Contents

PRIVATE AND CONFIDENTIAL?

Handling personal information in the social and health services

Edited by Chris Clark and Janice McGhee

This edition published in Great Britain in 2008 by

The Policy Press
University of Bristol
Fourth Floor
Beacon House
Queen's Road
Bristol BS8 1QU
UK

tel +44 (0)117 331 4054
fax +44 (0)117 331 4093
e-mail tpp-info@bristol.ac.uk
www.policypress.org.uk

British Library Cataloguing in Publication Data
A catalogue record for this book is available from the British Library.

Library of Congress Cataloging-in-Publication Data
A catalog record for this book has been requested.

ISBN 978 1 86134 905 7 paperback
ISBN 978 1 86134 906 4 hardcover

Cover design by Qube Design, Bristol.
Front cover: image kindly supplied by www.istockphoto.com
Printed and bound in Great Britain by Henry Ling Ltd, Dorchester.

Notes on contributors

Peter Ashe is an information consultant with NHS Scotland (National Services). He first published on 'Recording, ethics and data protection' in *New Information Technology in Management and Practice* (Horobin, G. and Montgomery, S. [eds], Kogan Page, 1986). As a member of the Association of Directors of Social Services Information Management Group (1983-2004) he contributed to most of the UK national initiatives in this area. He has worked locally on information sharing between health and social care since the early 1990s, leading the Scottish national eCare information sharing programme in its first, experimental, phase and being responsible for the early introduction of information sharing protocols between partner organisations. He began to develop the thinking underpinning his chapter while contributing to the development of a Scottish national Integrated Assessment Framework for all children.

Val Baker is Director of Clinical Information, NHS Lothian, Scotland. Previous experience in community nursing management and latterly as Head of Information Technology for an NHS Trust led to interest in the sharing of information and information governance in general. Her current post, which focuses on clinical engagement with a health strategy, includes senior responsibility for implementation of information governance standards in NHS Lothian. She has published a range of journal articles and is author of 'Information management and the use of technology' in *District Nursing: Providing Care in a Supportive Network* (Lawson, S., Cantrell, J. and Harris, J. [eds], Churchill Livingstone, 2000).

Cynthia Bisman is Professor of Social Work and Social Research at Bryn Mawr College in Pennsylvania, USA. Her extensive practice experience includes public welfare, severe mental illness, veterans, multi-problem families, supervision and organisational consultation. She has served as an ethics reviewer for the National Association of Social Workers. Her journal articles and books reflect her research interests in professional socialisation, development of practice theory and social work values and ethics. She contributes editorial functions for journals in the UK and US. She is currently using case material from recent interviews with social workers in the UK and US to infuse a values and social justice perspective in her revised edition of *Social Work Practice: Cases and Principles* originally published with Brooks/Cole in 1994.

Gary Clapton is Senior Lecturer in Social Work at the University of Edinburgh. His main interests are in adoption, child welfare, fathers and fatherhood and integration of student learning in social work. He is author of *Birth Fathers and their Adoption Experiences* (Jessica Kingsley, 2003) and *Relatively Unknown: A Year in the Life of the Adoption Contact Register for Scotland* (Family Care, 2003).

Chris Clark is Professor of Social Work Ethics and former Dean of Postgraduate Studies in the College of Humanities and Social Science at the University of Edinburgh. He is author of *Social Work Ethics: Politics, Principles and Practice* (Palgrave, 2000). His recent publications include articles on professional confidentiality, responsibility and moral character in social work.

Lisa Curtice is Director of the Scottish Consortium for Learning Disability (SCLD), which was set up to support implementation of *The Same as You?*, the Scottish government framework for services for people with learning difficulties in Scotland. Her main interests are user engagement, staff development, citizenship rights, health needs and personalised services. She is author of 'Listening and including people with learning disabilities' in *Learning Disability: A Handbook for Integrated Care* edited by Michael Brown (APS Publishing, 2003) and is a regular contributor to *Learning Disability Today*.

Lilian Edwards is an expert in family law and co-author of two editions of Edwards and Griffiths, *Family Law* (2nd edition, W. Green, 2006). She has taught family and child law in Scotland for almost 20 years and published widely in the area. She also specialises in Internet law, and is now Professor of Internet Law at the University of Southampton.

Ian Harper is Senior Lecturer in Social Anthropology at the University of Edinburgh. His interests are in medical anthropology, international health (particularly tuberculosis and infectious disease control), development and the Himalayas, particularly Nepal, and anthropological ethics. He has published articles on ethics and research in *Anthropology Today* and *Social Science and Medicine*, and on tuberculosis control and other public health issues in Nepal. He is presently researching as part of an interdisciplinary team on an ESRC/DfID-funded project on Tracing Pharmaceuticals in South Asia.

Susan Hunter is Lecturer in Social Work at the University of Edinburgh. Her most recent publication is *Co-production and Personalisation in Social Care* (co-edited with Pete Ritchie; Jessica Kingsley, 2007). She has extensive experience of chairing voluntary organisations with a record of innovation in the field of learning disability.

Hazel Kemshall is Professor of Community and Criminal Justice at DeMontfort University, Leicester. Formerly a probation officer, she has research interests in risk assessment and management of high-risk offenders, public protection and multi-agency work. She has published numerous articles and research reports, most recently *Understanding Risk in Criminal Justice* (Open University Press, 2003). She has extensively researched assessment and management practices with high-risk offenders, including for the Home Office, ESRC, Scottish Office and Scottish Executive.

Janice McGhee is Senior Lecturer in Social Work in the School of Social and Political Studies at the University of Edinburgh. She teaches both social work law and psychology and human development on the undergraduate and postgraduate social work programmes. Her main research interests are related to child welfare and protection and she has published extensively on the Scottish children's hearings system.

Rowena Rodrigues is a researcher in the School of Law at the University of Edinburgh. Her key research focus is digital identity and law. She has conducted extensive and in-depth research on data protection law and privacy, the legal implications of Radio Frequency Identification (RFID) and issues relating to wireless security. She has also researched and examined the working of the UK National DNA Database (NDNAD).

Ian E. Thompson was formerly Honorary Research Fellow at the University of Edinburgh and formerly Professor of Ethics and Philosophy at the University of Notre Dame Australia, Perth. His principal research interests are in professional and corporate ethics, healthcare and social policy, in competency-based training in ethics, in academic, professional and organisational contexts. His publications include *Nursing Ethics*, 5th edition (with Melia, K.M., Boyd, K.M. and Horsburgh, D; Elsevier, 2006) and *Responsible Management of Confidential Health Information* (with others; Health Department of Western Australia, 2002). He has also published research reports in public healthcare, social work, accounting and legal practice, as well as practice guidance resources for ethical management of public services including *Putting Ethics to Work in the Public Sector* (with Harries, M. and Vass, M.; Office of the Public Sector Standards Commission, 1997).

Jason Wood is Senior Lecturer in the Faculty of Health and Life Sciences at De Montfort University, Leicester. He has research interests and expertise in the community management of high-risk offenders, including the effectiveness of strategies used to involve the public. In 2005 he evaluated the implementation of Multi-Agency Public Protection Arrangements (MAPPA) with Kemshall and Mackenzie (Home Office, 2005). More recently, he led an investigation into MAPPA work with high-risk sex offenders (with Kemshall, Maguire, Hudson and Mackenzie) commissioned by the Home Secretary in 2006 for the Child Sex Offender Review (Home Office, 2007). He is currently completing his PhD in active citizenship and social policy.

Introduction

Janice McGhee and Chris Clark

Privacy and confidentiality are fundamental concepts in law, philosophy, anthropology, political theory, medicine, health and social welfare. They are also culture-specific, complex and problematic concepts in both theory and professional practice. Confidentiality is regarded as a central tenet of practice for medical, health, social work and other professionals in the health and personal social services. These professionals handle personal and often sensitive information obtained from the citizen as client, patient or service user. They do so with the primary intention of benefiting the individual's health and social welfare, and sometimes also with the aim of realising benefits for the wider society. Citizens have both legal and moral rights to assume that the information they disclose will not be shared without their consent; and where consent is given, that information shared will be limited in scope and restricted to personnel with relevant reasons for holding it.

Professional codes of ethics provide guidance and generally set out the basic principle of confidentiality. The legal framework (primarily encompassing the 1998 Data Protection Act, common law and the 1998 Human Rights Act) and administrative protocols provide for the further regulation of the management of personal information. Codes of ethics and the law do provide for situations where confidential information may justifiably be shared without consent. In daily practice applying professional codes and legislation is often fraught with these complex decisions, some of which may pose serious threats either to the rights of citizens or to the welfare of vulnerable individuals. There is a complex balance: central to decision making are questions of proportionality and necessity and how to balance legitimate public interest with rights to privacy.

Policy, organisational, legal and technological developments in health and social services provide a further set of complex challenges. The increasing emphasis on interprofessional and interagency working that policy requires for effective, 'joined-up' services presents new issues and dilemmas in preserving citizens' rights to confidentiality and privacy. In the context of the multidisciplinary team, citizens will consent to share information – but what are the limits on the nature and extent of the information shared and with whom, and how are these decisions best made? Where there are issues of individual capacity or understanding, what is the best way for these to be resolved to the benefit of the citizen?

Increasing accountability, legislative provisions and the necessity to share information to effectively provide integrated services have led to questioning of the traditional ideas of confidentiality often reflected in professional codes. In social work, Swain (2006) argues for a redefinition of the concept of confidentially in light of professional accountability at agency and governmental levels and legal frameworks that limit the extent of confidentiality available. He suggests instead a commitment to the respectful use of information, where possible with the agreement of the client, and within the legal framework. Hughes and Louw (2002) argue for a more sophisticated understanding of confidentiality, beyond very legalistic interpretations, in the context of multidisciplinary working with cognitively impaired patients. The patient with dementia is the shared concern of all the professionals and carers who are working together, and Hughes and Louw (2002, p 150) suggest that confidentiality here should not be the foremost principle but should best be seen as a 'token of respect and trust'.

The all-pervasive use of information and communication technology (ICT) and its impact on the ease and accessibility of information requires further examination. The rate of technological change is fast outpacing the systems and structures for managing personal information. The developing role of new technology is a theme resonating through many of the contributions to this book. There is a potential for new technology to drive policy and practice development because of its increasing power to scrutinise actions and gather and process information on citizens. The proliferation of electronic databases potentially allows for the greater monitoring of ever-larger swathes of the population. There are of course benefits to large-scale (anonymised) data gathering in supporting the strategic review and delivery of services; however, there is also significant potential for information to be used for purposes that are not covered by the original authority to gather data.

There are wide-ranging debates and analyses of the 'surveillance society' and of the role of new technology that cannot be addressed in detail here but provide an important background in considering the role of new technology in the health and personal social services. Wood in *A Report on the Surveillance Society* (2006) points out that surveillance of people is neither a new development nor the result of new technology (although this has enhanced capacity). It is seen to be part of day-to-day contemporary life in rich countries, reflected for example in supermarket loyalty cards and CCTV, and is a 'product of modernity'. He acknowledges there are benefits but also that large-scale systems present 'risks and dangers' and that 'power does corrupt or at least skews the vision of those who wield it' (p 1). The issue of trust is identified as central, while increasing surveillance in society, in the workplace and even within the family (referring to 'webcams and GPS systems' to monitor adolescents) serves to create suspicion and ultimately may damage social relationships. All this suggests that the increasing use of databases and new technology in health and social welfare needs to be examined beyond the usual questions around security and accuracy but also for the wider significance and unintended consequences that may arise.

It is clear therefore that privacy and confidentiality represent an increasingly challenging area of policy and practice where technological development, civil liberties, surveillance, health and welfare become inextricably intertwined. The contributors to this book reflect on central themes including the nature of confidentiality as a philosophical and culture-bound concept; questions of proportionality and necessity in balancing individual privacy with the public interest; the implications for those seen to have lesser autonomy in decisions to share information or not; the day-to-day policy and practice issues that arise in managing personal information; and the impact of new technology.

Professional confidentiality revisited

The book opens with a critical enquiry into basic principles of professional confidentiality and some of the difficulties it poses. Later parts go on to explore what the boundaries of confidentiality should be, since it is clear that while human flourishing generally is dependent on privacy there are also many occasions in which professionals have to intervene to infringe privacy precisely in order to protect the flourishing of vulnerable individuals.

Cynthia Bisman in Chapter One traces the classic grounds of confidentiality as an essential attribute of the professional relationship. Without confidentiality of what passes between the professional and the client there can be no privacy for the client. Privacy is necessary to safeguard individuals' basic moral right and psychological need for the protection of their autonomy. For this reason, a client's personal information should only be communicated to other parties with his (or her) informed and prior consent. Bisman particularly highlights that human flourishing or 'eudaimonia' depends on interpersonal relationships, and reminds us of the central place rightly given to the professional–client relationship in the founding period of modern social work. There seems to be a danger that the central focus on the professional relationship may be lost in contemporary social services. Bisman warns against professionals giving in to the pressures that currently threaten to erode privacy, autonomy and confidentiality.

Chris Clark in Chapter Two sets out to analyse a paradox presented by the theory of confidentiality in professional relationships. On the one hand, professionals are universally expected to demonstrate qualities of honesty, truthfulness and reliability in their dealings with clients, with each other and with the wider public. Nothing more quickly undermines trust in professionals than a perception that the advice on which we vitally depend might be intentionally distorted by half-truths or misrepresentations on the part of the professional. On the other hand, however, the ethic of professional confidentiality, designed as we have seen to shelter the privacy and enhance the autonomy of the individual, quite often seems to require professionals to be, at least, economical with the truth, and on occasion even to misrepresent the full truth in order precisely to protect confidentiality. Professionals thus seem to be bound by a double standard of truthfulness, which must be an absurdity. Drawing on recent theorising about truth-telling from philosophers MacIntyre and Williams, Clark proposes that professionals have to operate by what he terms a moderated or 'watchful' truthfulness, with professional confidentiality as a three-cornered contest of the professional's truthfulness towards the individual client, towards other people proximate to the client and towards the wider public good. Such a model serves to better understand the dilemmas that practitioners are expected to resolve on a daily basis while being obligated by unclear and frequently contradictory professional duties, rules and procedures.

In Chapter Three Ian Harper draws on his experience both as medical practitioner and anthropologist in Nepal to highlight the culturally specific nature of the Western idea of professional confidentiality – a discussion with obvious domestic implications for a multicultural society such as Britain. The conditions under which medical services operate in Nepal, as in many other developing countries, often do not practically permit the privacy for patients and clients that is routinely expected in the West and which, if not satisfied, becomes a point of censure by professional and regulatory bodies. More theoretically challenging, perhaps, is the observation that patients and their families do not expect, and perhaps do not want, the kind of confidentiality that is the norm in the West. In Nepal notions of patient privacy take second place to family and community solidarity. From health workers' point of view, moreover, the kind of solemn secrecy with which

HIV positive status is standardly guarded in the West may be seen as secondary to an expectation that community members need to be aware of a person's status, and to an expectation that professionals may need to break confidentiality in order to offer an individual treatment. Underlying such differences of service and practice are different concepts of individuality and community. Nevertheless, in academic social anthropology as in other spheres, the principles of protecting the autonomy of the individual, respecting confidentiality and ensuring informed consent remain paramount. Accepting that neither an agnostic cultural relativism, nor unquestioned reliance on the universal validity of Western moral and cultural norms, is a tenable position, Harper invites us to grapple with a set of issues that can only become more acute and pervasive with the growth of globalisation.

After his review of key principles and developments in the law and policy of professional confidentiality, Ian Thompson in Chapter Four applies his outlook as a philosopher to argue that defining workable and defensible practices for handling privacy and confidentiality is not best approached as an exercise in abstract moral theory or high-order policy. Instead, it should be developed in dialogue grounded in the real world of agencies and service practice. He suggests that the mystification of ethics as an abstract discipline has hindered the development of practical ethics for agency policy and professional practice. Thompson amplifies his argument with two contrasting case studies, one from Australia and the other from Scotland. In Western Australia an action research approach was adopted with practitioners and policy makers to develop agreed policies and procedures for the sharing and use of confidential health information. In the Outer Hebrides general issues were raised in the aftermath of an apparent child protection failure, which revealed inadequate record keeping and sharing and analysis of information. Thompson identifies some of the requisite tools, skills and methods useful for developing effective and accepted policies for protecting and sharing personal information at the ground level of service delivery.

Balancing individual privacy with the right to information

Balancing public interest and individual privacy rights is a longstanding and consistent theme in law and policy and is played out in the complex decisions professionals face in their day-to-day practice. There are boundaries on confidentiality and professionals sometimes have to intervene to infringe privacy to protect the welfare of other, often vulnerable, individuals. This is recognised in professional codes and the legal framework yet the boundaries of these decisions are not straightforward, not least because predicting individual risk is problematical.

Lilian Edwards and Rowena Rodrigues in Chapter Five provide a concise grounding in the essential concepts, international treaties and domestic legislation on which privacy, confidentiality and data protection are founded in law. 'Informational privacy' is now protected by the 1998 Data Protection Act, which is based on a right to privacy established by the European Convention on Human Rights. The concept of confidential communication, by contrast, is largely based in the common law, although it is rapidly being modified by developing ideas about individuals' right to privacy. The need for protection of privacy has become much more acute with the arrival of modern technology. Ubiquitous surveillance and the 'database society' allow unprecedented amounts of data to be stored, processed and cross-referenced; new safeguards are needed against unauthorised 'profiling' and 'data mining'; public policy must beware of 'fishing' for data for no particular purpose, and 'function creep', whereby data legitimately gathered for one purpose may start to be surreptitiously applied for other purposes. The authors go on to examine particularly the position of children in relation to informational privacy, where the right to privacy may need to be balanced against the need for protection and consideration of the child's capacity to give informed consent. Even when a child may be deemed competent to give consent, for example for medical treatment, there may still be circumstances in which the confidentiality of his (or her) communications may need to be broken without consent in order to protect against serious harm. Although it is well established that the public interest may occasionally require breaking confidentiality, professionals in social and health services must nevertheless recognise the danger of losing the child's trust or leaving the child in an even more vulnerable position. Edwards and Rodrigues conclude with an exploration of the complex issues raised by the prospect of a national database of all children, showing how children's rights to autonomy and privacy may be very difficult to reconcile with desirable parental consent, essential protection and possible wider public good. The implications of such a database are further explored by Ashe in Chapter Nine.

Public protection as a justification for reducing individual rights to privacy and confidentiality is explored in Chapter Six by Hazel Kemshall and Jason Wood in the context of multiagency arrangements to manage the risk serious sexual (and violent offenders) may present in the community, an area where political, public and media concern are to the fore. They indicate that public protection is the priority in exchanging information about offenders between agencies to assess and manage risk, and in disclosures to third parties who sometimes may be individual members of the public. The authors illustrate how the principles of necessity and proportionality are central to these decisions. The growing use of overt and covert surveillance, both human and technological, alongside restrictive measures (for example curfews) to manage risk is examined with 'community protection' potentially taking on the 'hallmarks of custody in the community'. All these features give rise to profound tensions in the balance between public protection, human rights and ethical considerations in the treatment of offenders who are the focus of much public fear and condemnation.

Gary Clapton in Chapter Seven begins from the fundamental need for all human beings to develop a sense of identity and the importance of knowledge of personal and family origins in this process. He discusses the policy, practice and attitudes that can restrict information for adopted people who seek access to adoption agency records. The chapter primarily discusses this issue in relation to the 'closed' adoptions of the 1950s–1970s – many of whose subjects are now seeking to trace their origins. Clapton illustrates how confidentiality for an agency and the birth parent(s) becomes a form of secrecy and gatekeeping for the adopted person seeking information. Despite changing attitudes towards adopted adults seeking information he argues that there are still 'powerful beliefs' that providing information on origins and adoptions may potentially be damaging. He reflects on the 'feelings of powerlessness' that can be engendered by the process of adoption and considers the view that the adopted adult remains treated or viewed as a child. This infantilisation of adopted adults is reflected in institutional practices and in the reality that the power to control information about oneself lies elsewhere. He makes a powerful argument for understanding and support for the adopted adult's search and for an open approach in practice to access despite issues of confidentiality, while recognising there may need to be forums for disputes to be resolved.

Working together

It is in the field of child protection, where the vulnerability and dependence of children requires that information be shared, that the issue of balance between state intervention and family autonomy is arguably most stark. Failures in communication and information sharing have been identified over many years in inquiries and reviews where children have died or been seriously injured in the context of abuse and neglect. In Chapter Eight Janice McGhee discusses the role of effective communication and information sharing to protect children at risk of abuse or neglect. She draws together a range of studies, inquiries and opinions to look beyond apparently straightforward critiques of poor practice in information sharing to some of the complexities in practice. McGhee considers the arguments for and against mandatory reporting laws as a potential solution to ensure that information is shared. The developing role of databases in this area is highlighted, and their potential to increase the surveillance of ever-larger numbers of children and their families.

The process of developing new rules and principles for sharing confidential client and patient information may be driven to a large extent by government policy initiatives, but it is practitioners on the ground who have to work out the new procedures and understandings that will enable information sharing to take place effectively while safeguarding individual rights. In Chapter Nine Peter Ashe draws on his personal experience as an adoptive parent as well as his professional role in the NHS to explore conceptual frameworks for sharing information in the world of children's services. He observes that children's policy has traditionally been divided between the realm of child protection, which focuses on the relatively small proportion of children at high risk and need, and the realm of education for the general population of children. What is emerging now is a tendency to extend the close planning and surveillance appropriate to child protection to the general population of children, with the consequent threat of unwarranted state control and invasion of privacy. At the same time, however, children and young people are exploring the unprecedented possibilities offered by 'Web 2.0' tools to take their own responsibility for developing their identity and setting the boundaries of privacy in the new public spaces of the Internet. Rather than addressing privacy and confidentiality solely on professionals' terms, policy will need to be increasingly responsive to where children are taking us. Moreover, both the policy process and planning at the level of the individual should be conceived as conversations conducted within a shared and enabling frame of reference – in contrast to conventional top-down social policy and paternalistic professional intervention.

Children, vulnerable adults and certain other groups in society are often seen to have more limited autonomy as compared with citizens in general, with consequent impact on their rights to privacy and self-determination. In Chapter Ten Susan Hunter and Lisa Curtice emphasise the importance of ensuring appropriate support to enable adults with learning disabilities to exercise their full citizenship rights and have greater control over their lives. They recognise that policy and practice have increasingly aimed to support individuals to have a greater say in controlling their lives, and they go on to explore a number of areas where tensions arise in balancing empowerment and protection. They critically discuss the use of technology and data sharing at service level and highlight tensions between data gathered to assess the benefits of service investment and the rights of individuals to express their opinions about the use of this information. Balancing the need to protect people with learning disabilities who are also 'vulnerable adults' is sharply brought into focus by the authors' discussion of the failure of health and social services to protect a woman with learning disabilities who was subject to prolonged physical and sexual abuse. The discussion of 'smart technology' explores benefits and concerns about capacity and consent and the potential for surveillance. Arguments of public interest and equity support research participation, and the need to improve research capacity to hear the often 'hidden voices' of people with profound disabilities is recognised. They conclude that, as with support and service improvement for people with learning disabilities, 'putting the person first' may be a better guiding light to the complexities of sharing information to the benefit of the individual.

Val Baker in Chapter Eleven offers a window into the fast-changing world of interagency information sharing in the 'Joint Future' of health and social services. Government has taken up the challenge to raise service standards right across the spectrum of service type and client need, and in this the effective sharing of relevant personal information about individuals is seen as critical. While the need for better information sharing is undoubtedly one of the key themes to emerge from inquiries into service failures over the past 30 years or more, the range of practical solutions potentially available has lately been revolutionised by the new, unprecedentedly powerful information technologies. What emerges therefore is a picture of pell mell change as government, agencies, professional bodies and practitioners constantly struggle to adopt new legislation and develop new information systems, tools and protocols, some of which seem destined for obsolescence almost before the website proclaiming them has been published. Echoing Thompson, experience reveals some marked contrasts of professional culture among the different professional groups who are increasingly expected to join up their respective areas of responsibility. Nevertheless, core principles for data sharing and data protection are gradually being elaborated and enhanced, based on the fundamental ethical standards of protection of privacy, informed consent and professional obligations to the wider public good.

Towards redefining the ethic of confidentiality

The contributors to this book offer a wide range of perspectives – philosophical, legal, social–scientific and professional – on the rapidly evolving expectations of confidentiality in the social and health services. The traditional ethic of professional confidentiality has been severely stretched, perhaps already to breaking point. How might we begin to redefine confidentiality in a way that conserves the core of human rights and privacy while addressing the widely agreed need to better share information for the benefit of individual clients, their kin and society as a whole?

The traditional ethic of professional confidentiality can be modelled as a set of relationships and expectations on three levels. Personal and private information belongs to the person it refers to – the individual human subject, whom we may conceive as the first or base level in the set of relationships governed by professional confidentiality. Individuals will, of course, make different choices about what they choose to reveal, and to whom; they have different conceptions of private space and private business; and these conceptions vary not only between individuals but also across social groups and cultures. In this book, Ian Harper (Chapter Three) illustrates the very different conceptions of individuality and privacy that may be found in different cultures. Nevertheless, the key principle embedded here (and reflected, for example, in the 1998 Data Protection Act) is that ownership of personal information belongs to the subject of the information. Cynthia Bisman (Chapter One) explores the importance of privacy to human flourishing, and its implications for professional ethics. Gary Clapton (Chapter Seven) shows that withholding personal information from adoptees negates their autonomy, and arguably in this way limits their individual flourishing.

At the second level is the professional who will deliberately gather personal information as part of the helping and service delivery process, and who will incidentally acquire other personal information that is not necessarily germane to the professional service but is nonetheless private. The professional therefore becomes the custodian of personal information and must maintain a relationship of trust with the owner of the information. This relationship of trust is both an ethical obligation stemming from the principle of respect, and a practical necessity for effective service delivery. All the contributors to this book have acknowledged the basis of trust that is essential to individuals' relationships with professionals.

At the third level are found the other professionals, their respective agencies and public authorities who need to receive and utilise the information that the original frontline professional has acquired in direct contact. As first custodian of the information, the frontline professional has to make daily judgements about what information about the client, patient or service user *may* be passed on to colleagues and what *must* be passed on; and equally, has to make discriminations about what *ought not* to be passed on and what *need not* be passed on. Many of the everyday dilemmas of professional practice over confidentiality turn on these issues. Many of the contributions to this book touch on the practical issues in sharing information between health and social services. McGhee (Chapter Eight) charts the complexities of information sharing in child protection, while Hunter and Curtice (Chapter Ten) reveal aspects of the complexity of the ownership of personal information in the case of adults with incapacity.

The key defining feature of this model is that the authority to use and communicate personal information is conceived as resting primarily with the individual client, patient or service user who is both the owner and subject of that information. The client and information owner chooses under certain circumstances to share information with a professional, who in effect is given a certain amount of licence to act on the individual's information. In turn, the professional makes certain choices about sharing the information with other members of the community, and with professionals or agencies, to whom a further portion of authority is thus devolved. This model therefore is hierarchical: authority to use personal information originates with the owner and client, and is progressively and partially handed down, by degrees, to the frontline professional and thence to other professionals, agencies and members of the community.

Notwithstanding its pervasiveness in professional codes of ethics, the contributions to this book cohere with the wider debate on personal information sharing in showing that this traditional, hierarchical three-level model has major deficiencies. Whatever its utility may have been for a possibly imaginary world of 19th-century professional practice, the model is plainly both inadequate as description and unsatisfactory as a guiding professional ethic for modern conditions. There are many different professional disciplines in the modern world of personal and health services, and they work within and across different service structures and organisations, but they must work together and not in isolation. The professions all explicitly recognise that their obligations to the client, patient or service user are not exclusive but must be balanced with wider obligations to other interested parties and to the public good. Government, too, is now expected to take a positive role in preventing harm and promoting social goods such as health and family flourishing. Such a role may be politically necessary and indeed widely welcomed, but it comes at a certain cost to the authority over personal information that is embedded in the traditional ethic of confidentiality.

Alongside these changes in politics and the professional role have arrived sweeping and unprecedented developments in the capacity to store, filter, collate and exchange information, making a daily reality of information sharing on a scale that was practically unimaginable only 20 years ago. The new technology puts enormous power into the hands of professionals and governments. Until recently the range of practical choices open to individuals was relatively little directly affected by governmental surveillance and corporate intelligence gathering, since information gathering about individual statuses and actions could only be selective in scope, sporadic in operation, weakly reliable, poorly analysed and little collated. Today's technology already makes the traditional picture of free choice in an open society highly questionable, even without the further major changes that are virtually certain in the immediate future. However, as Ashe illustrates in Chapter Nine, the shift of power is not just one way; the new technologies have already opened to the ordinary citizen information, choices and means of communication that were equally unimaginable 20 years ago.

If the old ethic of professional confidentiality is obsolescent, what is to replace it? The contributors to this book show that the conventional model of professional confidentiality as being decisively rooted in respect for individual autonomy is, in effect, only half the story. The other half of the story is that professionals and their organisations have wider obligations, to third parties and to the general good of the community. Professionals are accountable not only to the client but to a public mandate legitimated by a political process and exercised through accountable governance. Confidentiality for professionals and their clients is always and inherently a matter of balancing private interests and public good.

The chapters of this book adumbrate a new ethics of professional confidentiality that is now being worked out at ground level in service practice. This is a tentative, trial-and -error process, necessarily accompanied by much heartsearching lest the precious tradition of individual human rights should be lost sight of in the quest for service efficiency and better standards of welfare – and under the possible threat of governmental surveillance.

Effective systems of professional ethics have two essential components. The first essential is a set of agreed core values and principles. These are characteristically described in professional codes of ethics. Contemporary codes increasingly contain the intellectual resources necessary for working out the balance between private interests and public good. The second essential is an effective institutional framework for interpreting principles, determining cases, resolving conflicts, disciplining errant professionals and repairing faulty organisations. On this aspect the studies in this book show that there is still a long way to go, as professionals and their organisations struggle to master the complexities of interdisciplinary and interagency working in a world increasingly shaped by the new information technologies. We hope these studies will be a contribution to the ongoing work of theory, research and on-the-ground problem solving.

References

Hughes, J.C. and Louw, S.J. (2002) 'Confidentiality and cognitive impairment: professional and philosophical ethics', *Age and Ageing*, vol 31, no 2, pp 147-50.

Swain, P.A. (2006) 'A camel's nose under the tent? Some Australian perspectives on confidentiality and social work practice', *British Journal of Social Work*, vol 36, no 1, pp 91-107.

Wood, D.M. (ed) (2006) *A Report on the Surveillance Society for the Information Commissioner*, Surveillance Studies Network, www.ico.gov.uk/upload/documents/library/data_protection/practical_application/surveillance_society_full_report_2006.pdf

Part One
Professional confidentiality revisited

Personal information and the professional relationship: issues of trust, privacy and welfare

Cynthia Bisman

Summary

Philosophical, historical and political perspectives inform this chapter's exploration of the meaning and value of privacy in professional relationships. Rights of privacy allow for individual choice in deciding whether to share personal information with others. This provides individuals some control over the flow of information about themselves and confers on privacy a particular authority in protecting individual identity and sense of self. Grounding privacy and professional relationships within an ethical and moral framework clarifies how they contribute to social welfare and the social good. Virtue ethics can inform an understanding of privacy as a personal right and a public interest and allows us to see how professional relationships without privacy protections may exacerbate inequalities and oppression while rendering impossible the job of the professional. Relational theory and the ethics of caring are presented as some of the current instructive approaches to understanding professional relationships. Finally, the chapter emphasises the importance of confidentiality as a foundational component of professional relationships and discusses the responsibilities of professionals with respect to informed consent and autonomy.

Virtue ethics

Philosophy, in its engagement with meanings, offers deep insight into the components of a good life. We therefore turn to philosophers for guidance in elucidating the meanings of the main concepts in this chapter. Virtue ethics, initiated by Plato and furthered by his student Aristotle, encompasses ancient Greek beliefs about what constitutes a good life. Lodge (1950) points to the two levels of Plato's dialogues – individual and social. The former is materialist, valuing possessions, property and wealth. In contrast, concern in the social is for excellence and preservation of the community, power, law and order. Aristotle's description of political associations focuses on the ways in which societies create capacities for ethical practices and modes of existence.

Appiah (2003) is among a group of contemporary philosophers (Doris, 2002; Hursthouse, 2002; Sunstein, 2004) engaged in a re-examination of virtue ethics. Feminist philosophers (Brennan, 2002; Koggel, 2002; Sherwin, 2002) also contribute to the current dialogue by analysing the impact of different kinds of relationships on equality and oppression. This sense of the importance of virtue ethics is seen, as well, in the work of some of our best contemporary social scientists (Koocher and Keith-Spiegel, 1998; Dworkin, 2000; Banks, 2004; Hugman, 2005). All of these thinkers understand that virtues are not mere simple traits but complex and multilayered functions of self and of society. Accepting the complexity and context-sensitive nature of personal and public virtues is of particular importance for a meaningful consideration of what it means to achieve a state of 'eudaimonia'. Appiah (2006, p 8) clarifies:

> Aristotle presupposes that asking what it is to have a good life – and the Greek word he uses for 'life,' like ours, can mean both the period one is alive and what makes one a living thing – is the same as asking what it is to flourish, what it is to have what he called *eudaimonia*.

In his definitional shift away from Aristotle's emphasis on human nature, Appiah (2006, p 9) expands the meaning of eudaimonia:

> what it is for a person to flourish, and ... [what] we owe to other people ... how we ought to treat other people if we are to flourish ourselves; and how the ways in which we should treat other people depend on what it takes for them to flourish.

Pointing to a critical linkage between moral virtue and human flourishing, Appiah highlights the traditional virtues of prudence, justice, courage and compassion for their contribution to eudaimonia.

Here we are not concerned exclusively with what it takes for one to flourish but with whether individuals can and do facilitate others' flourishing. This contemporary understanding of virtue ethics grounds our examination of privacy and of professional relationships as we consider the moral accountability of social and health services to contribute to the social welfare – the flourishing of others – through the protection of privacy, confidentiality and informed consent.

Relational theory

Feminist philosophy, with its significant focus on relations, context and caring, is an important voice in moral philosophy. It reveals the importance of seeing 'persons ... as products of society, inseparable from the complex social interactions in which they engage' (Sherwin, 2002, p 294). From this perspective, one's ability to be a moral agent is defined by one's social connectedness. Eudaimonia thus expands to include individuals and their social environments since 'the pursuit of one's own flourishing cannot qualify as morally praiseworthy unless one is engaged ... in promoting the flourishing of an inclusive social collectivity' (Tessman, 2002, p 31).

In this framework 'relationships (professional and personal) are places where interactions can help or hinder a person's abilities to develop the capacities of rationality, autonomy and self-development' (Koggel, 2003, p 116) and we see how inequality is a form of oppression that must be addressed in the political and social realms. Koggel's argument furthers this position in equating relationship with achievement of equality, 'what it means to treat all people with equal concern and respect' (2002, p 250). Her challenge is to acknowledge that society actively sustains inequality, yet at the same time to expect a societal responsibility for making different social and policy choices to correct these inequalities. Furthermore, alleviation of oppression and enhancement of equality must cover a globally yet unequally connected human population. This is particularly necessary because the hierarchical structures in professional relationships can contribute to continuing and deepening oppression even as the subordination becomes less and less visible (Isaacs, 2002).

Social relations are important for identity formation and values clarification and have 'moral and political significance in relationships of oppression and privilege between groups' (Sherwin, 2002, p 289). Speech is also relational and as such can be limited or constrained by the power dynamics in relationships as well as social policies and practices. Koggel's (2003) analysis offers a compelling explanation of the significance of speech in self-development and autonomy and recaptures earlier arguments by Mill (1859) that public and open discussion of ideas is an essential communal process as it provides the only means for arriving at truth. This argument also builds on Sherwin's (2002) view by distinguishing the traditional liberal view of speech as abstract from a more nuanced understanding of the various relationship contexts in which utterances are made and thus define the speaker and the social and political realms. As Buber (1970) states, 'relation is reciprocity ... my You acts on me as I act on it' (p 67); 'all actual life is encounter' (p 62). Seen in this way, relationships allow 'for understanding the ways in which speech always has the potential to do harm or good for people living in the context of unequal opportunities, status, and levels of power' (Koggel, 2003, p 120).

To guard against the use of private relationships as a source or continuation of political and social inequality, Koggel (2003) advocates state protection, noting that as 'the therapeutic relationship would be viewed as a vehicle for addressing inequalities in the private lives of its citizens, state protection of privacy would be understood as promoting equality' (p 117). Again, this argument echoes Mill's linkages between persons and their environments; equality is a matter of justice and a means for improving man (as Mill would put it), while environment is influential in forming the character of man. Man and government shape each other. Every governmental action or inaction benefits certain people and disadvantages other people; societal progress and social welfare require governmental protection of privacy rights in professional relationships (Kurer, 1991).

For feminist moral philosophers there are ethical issues of character and trust. Sherwin (1992) points to the negative effects that lying has on relationships, with the compounding difficulties in the development of trust, character, individual development and responsibility. Her conceptualisation, similar to Koggel's above, is that the relationships women have with each other are essential in their emancipation. It is important here to note that in professional relationships in health and social welfare, women tend to outnumber men both as service providers and recipients. This places women in positions of increasing the oppression of other women, adding to the inequality of both groups.

Buber also emphasises the centrality of social relatedness of humans and believes conflicts arise from the relations of individual to community. 'The structures of communal human life derive their life from the fullness of the relational force that permeates their members' (Buber, 1970, p 98).

Although Buber believes the 'I-Thou' is the supreme human relationship, he acknowledges that such experiences are quite rare. The 'I-Thou' is dialogic; its emphasis on persons and interpersonal relationships allows for responsibility in life, 'man becomes an I through a You' (1970, p 80). The essence of life is personal relationships and knowledge of oneself is inherently knowledge of self in relation to others, '... the actual and fulfilled present exists only insofar as presentness, encounter and relation exist. Only as the You becomes present does presentness come into being' (1970, p 61).

Human contact in the professional relationship

The root of the word 'profess' is to take vows, to accept a calling. Professionals are *called* to their work by a moral commitment to serve the community and the greater good. Service to society, shaped by a profession's values and ethics, is the feature that most distinguishes professions. Professions require a commitment to ends to be served and not just the techniques practised (Lubove, 1977; Howe, 1980). The service is not only to the individual clients, but to the welfare of the society, to 'a larger whole, to a larger good of the community' (Gustafson, 1982, p 512). Early in social work's history, Kellogg recognised the relationship of social welfare and individual welfare: 'social evils are whatever things work against the common welfare of men. Society is a unit – a solidarity, of which individuals are a part. The person gains his highest development in that unity' (cited in Pumphrey and Pumphrey, 1961, p 176).

From its beginnings social work recognised the centrality of relationship in the form of 'friendly visitors' who gave alms to the poor. Richmond (1899, p 80) explained friendly visiting as 'intimate and continuous knowledge of and sympathy with a poor family's ... entire outlook on life'. During these visits, relationship was to function as 'mind over mind' to help clients further their own best interests (Richmond, 1922, p 102). Relationship was further emphasised in one of the early US social work conferences: 'the flesh and blood is in the dynamic relationship between the social caseworker and the client ... to achieve the fullest possible development of his personality (AASW, 1929, p 29). More recently, Bisman (1994, pp 77-8) defines relationship as a belief 'through which the client develops self-worth and trust in the competence of the social worker' and considers it 'the medium for social workers and client to connect together ... to help the client create change of self and of circumstance'.

The centrality of the professional relationship in social work is a feature equally shared by other professions. Martin (2000) interprets professional ethics across a wide range of professions, including medicine, law and religious ministry, as more than a matter of sticking to the rules and dealing with occasional dilemmas. Professionalism is rather to be understood as a commitment to certain personal commitments and ideals, indeed as a way of life. In his discussion of caring about clients, Martin (2000, p 69) explains that '[c]aring about persons, in a sense that refers to motives and attitudes as well as conduct, permeates the meaning-giving commitments that sustain professionals throughout demanding careers'.

According to the traditional view, trust in the professional's competence and expertise is the basis on which clients concede to professionals a *monopoly of judgement*, as 'professionals profess to know better the nature of certain matters, to know better than their clients what ails them' (Lynn, 1963, p 2). There are those who believe that increasing emphasis on specialisation may decrease attention to the moral component of the social ends professions serve (Brint, 1994), and some argue for new practice spaces to increase participation by service users, reduce hierarchy and promote equality (Burkett and McDonald, 2005). Managerialism and emphasis on evidence-based services may continue to alter not only the nature of relationship in the professional context but also the role and function of professional services.

Despite varying perspectives about their nature, professional relationships continue to be distinguished by use of human contact as a vehicle for creating change in conditions such as illness, social disorder, oppression, inequality, discrimination, injustice, child abuse or neglect. Professions, it is argued, have public protection and sanction because of their base in a moral function that benefits communities, the public, clients and the common good (see Bisman, 2004, for fuller discussion). As Tawney (1948, pp 94-5) states, the meaning of action in the context of the professional relationship, for professionals and the public, is 'that they make health, or safety ... or good law'.

It is through the medium of the professional relationship that individual and social change is implemented. Relationships in social work target 'social change, ... and the empowerment and liberation of people to enhance well-being' (BASW, 2002, p 1). The core function of social workers is to promote social justice and the alleviation of oppression with an emphasis on human well-being (Austin, 1983; Leiby, 1984; NASW, 1996; IFSW, 2004).

Confidentiality and privacy

Professional relationships and responsible practice are guided by each profession's overarching mission of service to a larger social good. The usually abstract concepts of a mission, such as social work's promotion of social justice, become more specific, distinct and less amorphous via a set of values and a code of ethics. All the same, greater specificity may not always increase clarity. As Bersoff (2003, p 155) states: '[e]xcept for the ultimate precept – above all, do no harm – there is probably no ethical value in psychology that is more inculcated than confidentiality.... Yet, there is probably no ethical duty more misunderstood'. Daniel and Kitchener (2000, p 78) explain confidentiality as a 'commitment made by a professional that non-public information will not be disclosed to a third party without consent'.

Wilson (1978), in one of the earliest books on confidentiality in social work, explains that confidentiality confers a duty on professionals to not speak about certain matters. She distinguishes this duty from a privilege, which is governed by law and belongs to the patient. Koocher and Keith-Spiegel (1998) concur that confidentiality is a standard of professional conduct as distinct from privilege, which is a legal protection. In order to practise ethically and without violating any laws, professionals need to appreciate this distinction between privilege and duty. Confidentiality as a privilege in the legal sense may at times belong to the client or the professional – in that either may have the privilege to divulge or not divulge certain details outside of the context of the relationship – whereas a duty to divulge or not divulge is an obligation, albeit a moral as well as a legal one, almost always imposed primarily and sometimes exclusively on the professional, the breaking of which carries moral and legal, as well as practical/functional, consequences.

Ideally, confidentiality allows individuals to talk about difficulties and possible solutions at reduced risk of incurring harm (for example, curtailment of healthcare, prosecution under the law, ridicule or social alienation) and allows for research that would otherwise be difficult (for example, into antisocial behaviour). One of the basic tenets of confidentiality is that knowledge acquired during the professional relationship must be used solely for the purposes of the professional interaction and protection of the client's interests. Confidentiality allows for disclosure and self-reflection, which in turn promote moral and intellectual development and autonomy; 'the protection of confidentiality is one vehicle for creating relationships that enable free speech and promote self-development' (Koggel, 2003, p 121).

In the context of the professional relationship, the person being served must relinquish some measure of privacy for the professional to be able to assess the situation and provide aid. It is the relinquishment of privacy in sharing personal information integral to one's identity that requires confidentiality, as 'individuals ought to have the freedom to shape their own interests, projects, and goals without interference from other individuals or the state' (Koggel, 2003, p 113). Sharing highly personal and intimate details of one's life is usually difficult, albeit necessary for the benefits of the helping relationship; confidentiality provides safety for this beneficial and limited relinquishment of privacy.

The dynamic of the confessional booth and practice within the 'Hippocratic Oath' have shaped an understanding of confidentiality that enables individuals to talk openly about information that would otherwise not be easily shared. Confidentiality facilitates the cooperation by patients that is needed 'in order for treatment to work' (Levin et al, 2003, p 2). Weak or inconsistent protection of privacy rights limits openness in these relationships, forces the professional to engage in piecemeal guesswork, and ultimately places an even more unmanageable burden on persons in need of help because they are already in a fragile or vulnerable situation. The core point is that without strong protection of confidentiality, the person who needs help cannot trust the professional and thus may not disclose crucial private details necessary to receiving any real help.

Arguing that weakened confidentiality requirements in these already unequal relationships can lead to further oppression in the lives of disadvantaged people, Koggel (2003, p 121) calls for expanding privacy from an individual to a social right because 'access to the personal records of patients who are members of traditionally disadvantaged groups entrenches rather than alleviates inequalities', and it is 'society's responsibility to prevent the harm of ... those who are most vulnerable...'. Bisman and Hardcastle (1999) agree that the protection of confidentiality cannot rest solely on utilitarian grounds but must be grounded in the deontological rationale that individuals have basic inalienable rights and that among these rights are by necessity the right to privacy and the right to be secure from harm. Denike (2000) advocates for policies that cultivate social equality and support vulnerable populations. Bell (1992) and Tessman (2002) share these concerns, pointing to the potential destructive effects of disclosure of confidential information on psychosocial functioning as well as increasing discrimination in housing, employment, education and healthcare.

Tensions around confidentiality are not new. In her early book on social work practice, Richmond (1917) pointed to its importance, despite pressures by a group called the Confidential Exchange (a misnomer), established to avoid duplication of services. During the present era shifts from rights to interests have increased the power of legislators in decisions about when to divulge or withhold information (Daniel and Kitchener, 2000). From the *technological* advances of recent decades we see a contracting or restricting of certain *legal* privacy protections that have led to an expansion of use of people's personal information for financial gain (by insurance companies, healthcare providers and banks, among others). The problem is now so serious that privacy protection in certain contexts such as credit cards, travel and banking is scarcely credible. The technological and legal landscapes in those contexts should definitely not serve as a model for how we address privacy and confidentiality in professional relationships in, for example, healthcare or social work or legal services. The relationship between a bank and a customer is of a categorically different nature than the relationship between professional and a client. Whatever protections may be available via technological empowerment to the bank customer are, by the very nature of the relationship, not available to a person who is in need of professional help.

Yeo and Brock (2003) point out that easier access to and use of personal information, made possible by technology and computerisation, induces an ever-increasing demand by service providers for more health information, as well as access to criminal histories and financial records. As it becomes easier to access previously confidential personal information, service providers may understand less well the dangers of accessing and using this information. Thus the basic assumptions underlying the professional relationship change and it may become impossible for the service provider, now addicted to this ease of access to so much information about often nameless/faceless clients, to respect client confidentiality and the nature of the professional relationship. Demands for breaking confidentiality include pressures such as audits, evidence-based practices and cost-benefit modelling. Brint (1994) also worries that technological changes may continue to diminish our understanding of the traditional meaning and value of confidentiality in professional relationships. Reamer (2000) raises the issue of inadvertent disclosures (such as answering machines and cell phones) as well as disclosures resulting from worker impairment such as substance abuse or mental health difficulties. We need ways to minimise the ripple effects associated with these disclosures – such as a duty to immediately communicate an unauthorised disclosure to the client and regulatory authority.

Informed consent and autonomy

While 'confidentiality is the practical outcome of valuing freedom and autonomy in a liberal society' (Koggel, 2003, p 113), informed consent is a means to protect privacy and a precondition for autonomy. Freeman

(1975, p 32) explains that there is 'a positive right of informed consent which exists both in therapeutic and experimental settings.... From whence derives the right? It arises from the right each of us possesses to be treated as a person'. Moreover, autonomy encourages critical reflection and individual responsibility. Dworkin (1988, p 90) offers the following perspective:'consent preserves the autonomy of the individual because his right to self-determination, his control of his body and his possessions, can be abrogated only with his agreement'. Principles that guide professional practice include written consent to release information to others, client access to information and records and warnings of potential risks. Codes of practice refer to self-determination and empowerment as the ethical basis for informed consent'(Bisman and Hardcastle, 1999).

Informed consent in healthcare developed in the context of injury claims. The US Federal Privacy Act of 1974 defined informed consent as the 'knowing consent of an individual or his legally authorised representative, so situated so as to be able to exercise free power of choice without undue inducement, ... constraint or coercion' (Federal Privacy Act, 1974). The ruling by Justice Cardozo in a seminal US Supreme Court decision – 'every human being of adult years and sound mind has a right to determine what shall be done with his own body' – still shapes legal decisions (*Schloendorff v Society of New York Hospital*, (1914) 211 N.Y. 125). Yet, the meaning of 'so situated so as to be able to exercise free power of choice' is not clear. Who decides whether someone is an adult of sound mind? What are the standards? How do we deal with evolving standards? Responses to these questions are influenced by continually shifting societal norms.

The principles of liberty and autonomy continue to drive our discussion. Initiated by the Greek city–state, autonomy refers to a kind of self-rule in which citizens can, in certain areas of life, make their own laws. To attain the level of equality required for self-rule and for functioning democracies, citizens must necessarily be independent moral agents. Shared by philosophers as diverse as Royce (1908), Sartre (1956) and Wolff (1973) is the conviction that moral agents are necessarily autonomous. Dworkin (1988, pp 80-1) postulates an intrinsic value 'to being able to make choices. What makes a life *ours* is that it is shaped by our choices, is selected from alternatives'. Autonomy's significant role in moral theory is partly a function of its weak content. What makes an individual particular is this pursuit of autonomy, the 'construction of meaning in his life.... It is because other persons are creators of their own lives ... that their interests must be taken into account, their rights protected' (Dworkin, 1988, p 110).

Mill further illuminates this discussion with his writings about liberty. The 'sole end … in interfering with liberty … is self-protection … the only purpose for which power can be rightfully exercised over any member of a civilized community, against his will, is to prevent harm to others' (Mill, 1859, p 223). This line of reasoning supports the duty to protect principle discussed in the previous section on confidentiality. Mill (1972, p 178) further states that 'human beings are only secure from evil at the hands of others in proportion as they have the power of being, and are, self-protecting'.

Berlin's (1984) framework of rights and liberty also addresses autonomy, which he equates with dignity, integrity, equality, individuality, responsibility and self-knowledge – all of which are desirable. For Berlin, the primary issue is personal freedom over state tyranny with one central question: '[b]y whom am I to be governed?' (1984, p xlvii). Berlin frames freedom of speech as a negative right: society should allow no or only extremely minimal governmental action limiting the right. With regard to positive rights, however, Berlin sees a need for substantial governmental support. A good example is education, where access for all citizens requires oversight and funding (1984). Drawing from this tradition, Koggel reminds us that in liberal theory, negative rights have priority, because of the greater importance in a liberal society on 'what the state must *refrain from doing* to maximize individual freedom', rather than what it can provide in the realm of positive rights (2003, p 115; emphasis original).

By contrast, from a relational theory perspective autonomy is reframed by Sherwin as dependent on interconnections between individual choices and the social context in which they are made, 'the social conditions that support – or inhibit – each person's ability to identify and pursue her own concerns' (Sherwin, 2002, p 290). To address the paradox for feminist agency that Isaacs believes is inherent in traditional views of agency (that is, that women may not attain certain standards of independence and choice), she proposes to 'think of the self-in-relation … in terms of the possibilities for action that being a self-in-relation creates' (Isaacs, 2002, p 137). This reformulation of agency shifts from the traditional individualistic emphasis to a care-based agency and may be germane for men as well as women.

The point is that no one has unrestrained agency or unrestricted privacy. Some constraints on autonomy are necessary and in these situations, informed consent provides a means of protecting autonomy. To assure such protection, Buchanan (1978) suggests certain guidelines for determining when constraining individual autonomy may be most acceptable or justifiable. The interest of the majority must be evident, the pain on the minority limited, and the costs high without the restraints. Contemporary problematic situations that would benefit from guidelines include civil commitment when an individual is a danger to self or others or incarceration when an individual has violated a society's laws or norms. Many urban areas in the US (including New York City, Philadelphia and Detroit) face continuing struggles with policies to move homeless persons into shelters when the temperature drops below freezing.

The possibility of consent by proxy arises when individuals cannot, or will not or should not, provide consent. These situations include, among others, persons who have mental impairment or are minors. Essential to such consent, in which autonomy is negated, is representation of the individual's interest. In such cases the nature of the representation becomes critical and this raises important questions around who is authorised to make decisions and under what criteria. Acting in the place of the person represented, the proxy must aim to perceive **his (or her)** wishes and best interests. Pitkin (1969) recommends that such consent should preserve what any rational person would want and consider what the incompetent person might choose. When professionals substitute their judgement for that of the client, Buchanan believes they run the risk of treating clients as less than moral equals. The conditions under which such substitutions occur require 'a critical examination of justifications' (1978, p 390). Professionals may justify such behaviour as an effort to promote the client's benefit, but it may well be a breach of codes of practice in that it violates self-determination and interferes with another's autonomy and liberty.

Reamer (2001) explains that due to court decisions, regulations and growing emphasis on the ethical code, understanding and protecting the right of informed consent in the US is increasingly important. Wise and minimal use of proxy consent and strict attention to informed consent is necessary to protect the autonomy of the professional as well as the client. He suggests the following elements relevant to research and evaluation: no coercion, ascertaining the competence of the participant, obtaining consent for specific procedures, and the right to refuse or withdraw consent.

In the previous section of this chapter the right to privacy and thus confidentiality was presented as inalienable. There are circumstances in which clients should not, even if in a position to give informed consent, be allowed to abdicate the right to privacy. Equally, there are also circumstances in which no amount of information giving can be presumed sufficient for a basis of informed consent, such as when dealing with a minor, or a person of limited mental capacity, or an adult in a state of shock or in a delusional state. In such circumstances, if there is no trustee or if that person is not available, the professional must assume the role of trustee and, regardless of the potential for rebuke by the hiring organisation, must not presume the client to be capable of being informed enough to be able to consent. Professionals must be diligent and resist pressure that will reduce informed consent and autonomy.

Conclusion

Attention to and respect for the flourishing of all persons must guide policy and practice in social and health services. Appiah's (2006, p 9) definition of eudaimonia – 'how we ought to treat other people if we are to flourish ourselves; and how the ways in which we should treat other people depend on what it takes for them to flourish' – and the resurgent interest in virtue ethics, offer guidance for understanding professional relationships, privacy and informed consent. Similarly, the philosophical traditions that focus on how liberty, autonomy and freedom constitute a good life should inform our contemporary understanding of the fundamental nature of the right to privacy and confidentiality in the context of the professional relationship.

Moral agency is a prerequisite to the flourishing of a people. Although Berlin (1984, p 10) advises that 'autonomy functions as a moral, political and social ideal' (1984, p 10), it is an ideal that demands continual vigilance and our eternal seeking because 'a genuine political community must ... be a community of independent moral agents' (Dworkin, 1996, p 26). In contemporary society self-determination may well be an illusion, but as Perlman (1971, p 125) admonishes, it 'is one of the "grand illusions" basic to human dignity and human freedom'. Mill (1859), in his defence of liberty, emphasises that people should be actively involved in deliberations about their own lives as players, and in fact as the key actor. Taking responsibility for one's life requires choice, action and courage to engage in the real world, yet as we have seen, societal protections are paramount.

Consequently, societal valuing of autonomy is a necessary condition for eudaimonia; the ability to make choices, a prerequisite for being a moral individual, depends on informed consent. 'A person's basic needs are the things required to avoid impairment of the ability to have values for one's life ... they are requirements of a life that is autonomous' (Copp, 2001, p 203). In addition to civil and social liberties and freedom from interference by state and other individuals, autonomy requires protection of privacy. Violations of the right to privacy threaten the autonomy of both clients and professionals. Hence, this argument encompasses protection of confidentiality in its protection of privacy and negative liberty.

Pressures on professionals to weaken the liberal and democratic foundations of the right to privacy, autonomy and confidentiality threaten to further commodify professions, as decisions are increasingly driven by market conditions rather than the needs of the client and the serving professional. Relational approaches, with their emphasis on the impact of political and social contexts on private and public relationships, provide critical perspectives on the potential oppressive effects of power and inequality in professional relationships affected by class, race and gender. We must place a heavy burden on relationships as the defining feature of professional occupations. To achieve their ends of moral and intellectual development, professional relationships rely on the trustworthiness of the professional to protect the client's right to privacy and informed consent. The divulging of private information corrupts everyone in a society, with particular peril for the most vulnerable populations. Public support of the right to privacy requires an inclusive definition of community membership accompanied by equal protection of all.

Implications of weakened privacy protections may be increased oppression and injustice, with a corresponding decrease in social welfare and negative effects on the flourishing of professionals as well as the clients they serve. Continuing questions include: Who will make decisions about privacy and under what criteria? How will societies protect oppressed or vulnerable groups such as women, people from black and minority ethnic communities, gays and lesbians, disabled people and those in poverty? If autonomy is a moral good should we not guard against its loss? How critical to social welfare is the freedom to choose? In this more market-driven era, what is the role of virtue ethics in policy and practice decisions?

Technological growth will likely continue at its current exponential pace, pressing health and social services towards ever-greater sharing of information, including information that should be private and confidential. The moral stance argued here will be increasingly needed to safeguard the basic core values of professional disciplines, protect individuals' rights to privacy and nourish what will otherwise be a waning orientation to social welfare. Regardless of our technological abilities, our society needs to reground the professional relationship and the protections surrounding this relationship in its proper moral and functional legal framework. The existence of a liberal society along with its social professions depends on it.

References

AASW (American Association of Social Workers) (1929) *Social Casework – Generic and Specific*, New York: AASW.

Appiah, K.A. (2003) *Thinking it Through: An Introduction to Contemporary Philosophy*, Oxford: Oxford University Press.

Appiah, K.A. (2006) Flexner lectures at Bryn Mawr College, November, Unpublished.

Austin, D. (1983) 'The Flexner myth and the history of social work', *Social Service Review*, vol 57, no 3, pp 357-77.

Banks, S. (2004) *Ethics, Accountability and the Social Professions*, Basingstoke: Palgrave.

BASW (British Association of Social Workers) (2002) *The Code of Ethics for Social Work*, Brighton: BASW.

Bell, N. (1992) 'Women and AIDS', in H. Holmes and L. Purdy (eds) *Feminist Perspectives in Medical Ethics*, Bloomington, IN: Indiana University Press, pp 46-62.

Berlin, I. (1984) *Four Essays on Liberty*, Oxford: Oxford University Press.

Bersoff, D. (2003) *Ethical Conflicts in Psychology* (3rd edition), Washington, DC: American Psychological Association.

Bisman, C. (1994) *Social Work Practice: Cases and Principles*, Pacific Grove, CA: Brooks Cole.

Bisman, C. (2004) 'Social work values: the moral core of the profession', *British Journal of Social Work*, vol 34, no 1, pp 109-23.

Bisman, C. and Hardcastle, D. (1999) *Integrating Research into Practice: A Model for Effective Social Work*, Pacific Grove, CA: Brooks Cole.

Brennan, S. (ed) (2002) *Feminist Moral Philosophy*, Calgary: University of Calgary Press.

Brint, S. (1994) *In an Age of Experts*, Princeton, NJ: Princeton University Press.

Buber, M. (1970) *I and Thou*, New York: Charles Scribner's and Sons.

Buchanan, A. (1978) 'Medical paternalism', *Philosophy and Public Affairs*, vol 7, no 4, pp 370-90.

Burkett, I. and McDonald, C. (2005) 'Working in a different space: linking social work and social development', in I. Ferguson, M. Lavalette and E. Whitmore (eds) *Globalisation, global justice and social work*, London: Routledge, pp 173-87.

Copp, D. (2001) *Morality, Normativity, and Society*, Oxford: Oxford University Press.

Daniel, P. and Kitchener, K. (2000) 'Confidentiality: doing good, avoiding harm, and maintaining trust', in K. Kitchener (ed) *Foundations of Ethical Practice, Research, and Teaching in Psychology*, London: Lawrence Erlbaum, pp 77–110.

Denike, M. (2000) 'Credibility and feminist legal strategy', Paper presented at the conference on the feminine principle, University of Texas at Arlington.

Doris, J. (2002) *Lack of Character: Personality and Moral Behaviour*, Cambridge: Cambridge University Press.

Dworkin, G. (1988) *The Theory and Practice of Autonomy*, Cambridge: Cambridge University Press.

Dworkin, R. (1996) *Freedom's Law: The Moral Reading of the American Constitution*, Cambridge, MA: Harvard University Press.

Dworkin, R. (2000) *Sovereign Virtue: The Theory and Practice of Equality*, Cambridge, MA: Harvard University Press.

Federal Privacy Act of 1974, US Public Law 93-579, enacted 31 December 1974, effective 27 September 1975, *Federal Register*, Part V-VI (8 October 1975).

Freeman, B. (1975) 'A moral theory of consent', *Hastings Center Report*, August, p 32.

Gustafson, J. (1982) 'Profession as callings', *Social Service Review*, vol 56, no 4, pp 501-5.

Howe, E. (1980) 'Public professions and the private model of professionalism', *Social Work*, vol 25, no 3, pp 179-91.

Hugman, R. (2005) *New Approaches to Ethics for the Caring Professions*, Basingstoke: Palgrave.

Hursthouse, R. (2002) *On Virtue Ethics*, Oxford: Oxford University Press.

IFSW (International Federation of Social Workers) (2004) *Code of Ethics*, Switzerland: IFSW.

Isaacs, T. (2002) 'Feminism and agency', in S. Brennan (ed) *Feminist Moral Philosophy*, Calgary: University of Calgary Press, pp 129-54.

Koggel, C. (2002) 'Equality analysis in a global context: a relational approach', in S. Brennan (ed) *Feminist Moral Philosophy*, Calgary: University of Calgary Press, pp 247-72.

Koggel, C. (2003) 'Confidentiality in the liberal tradition: a relational critique', in C. Koggel, A. Furlong and C. Levin (eds) *Confidential Relationships*, Amsterdam: Rodopi Press, pp 113-31.

Koocher, G. and Keith-Spiegel, P. (1998) *Ethics in Psychology* (2nd edition), Oxford: Oxford University Press.

Kurer, O. (1991) *John Stuart Mill: The Politics of Progress*, London: Garland Publishing.

Leiby, J. (1984) 'Charity organization reconsidered', *Social Service Review*, vol 58, no 4, 523-38.

Levin, C., Koggel, C. and Furlong, A. (2003) 'Questions and themes', in C. Koggel, A. Furlong and C. Levin (eds) *Confidential Relationships*, Amsterdam: Rodopi Press, pp 1-9.

Lodge, R. (1950) *Plato's Theory of Ethics*, London: Routledge & Kegan Paul.

Lubove, R. (1977) *The Professional Altruist: The Emergence of Social Work as a Career, 1880-1938*, New York: Atheneum.

Lynn, K. (1963) *The Professions in America*, Boston, MA: Houghton-Mifflin.

Martin, M. W. (2000) *Meaningful Work: Rethinking Professional Ethics*, New York: Oxford University Press.

Mill, J. S. (1859) 'On liberty', in J. M. Robson (ed) *Collected Works of John Stuart Mill*, vol 18, Toronto: Toronto University Press, pp 213-310.

Mill, J. S. (1972) *Considerations on Representative Government in Three Essays*, Oxford: Oxford University Press.

NASW (National Association of Social Workers) (1996) *Code of Ethics*, Washington, DC: NASW.

Perlman, H. (1971) *Perspectives on Social Casework*, Philadelphia, PA: Temple University Press.

Pitkin, H. (1969) *Representation*, New York: Atherton.

Pumphrey, R. and Pumphrey, M. (1961) *The Heritage of American Social Work*, New York: Columbia University Press.

Reamer, F. (2000) 'Ethical issues in direct practice', in P. Allen-Meares and C. Garvin (eds) *The Handbook of Direct Social Work Practice*, Thousand Oaks, CA: Sage Publications, pp 589-610.

Reamer, F. (2001) 'Ethical issues', in B. Thyer (ed) *The Handbook of Social Work Research Methods*, Thousand Oaks, CA: Sage Publications, pp 429-44.

Richmond, M. (1899) *Friendly Visiting among the Poor*, New York: Macmillan.

Richmond, M. (1917) *Social Diagnosis*, New York: Russell Sage Foundation.

Richmond, M. (1922) *What is Social Casework? An Introductory Description*, New York: Macmillan.

Royce, J. (1908) *The Philosophy of Loyalty*, New York: Macmillan.

Sartre, J. P. (1956) *Being and Nothingness: An Essay on Phenomenological Ontology*, trans H.E. Barnes, New York: Philosophical Library..

Sherwin, S. (1992) 'Feminist medical ethics: two different approaches to contextual ethics', in H. Holmes and L. Purdy (eds) *Feminist Perspectives in Medical Ethics*, Bloomington, IN: Indiana University Press, pp 17–31.

Sherwin, S. (2002) 'The importance of ontology for feminist policy-making', in S. Brennan (ed) *Feminist Moral Philosophy*, Calgary: University of Calgary Press, pp 273–95.

Sunstein, C. R. (2004) 'Moral heuristics and moral framing', *Minnesota Law Review*, vol 88, no 6, p 1556.

Tawney, R. H. (1948) *The Acquisitive Society*, New York: Harcourt Brace.

Tessman, L. (2002) 'On not living the good life: reflections on oppression, virtue and flourishing', in S. Brennan (ed) *Feminist Moral Philosophy*, Calgary: University of Calgary Press, pp 3–32.

Wilson, S. (1978) *Confidentiality in Social Work*, New York: Free Press.

Wolff, R. (1973) *The Anatomy of Reason*, New York: Harper and Row.

Yeo, M. and Brock, A. (2003) 'The moral framework of confidentiality and the electronic panopticon', in C. Koggel, A. Furlong and C. Levin (eds) *Confidential Relationships*, Amsterdam: Rodopi Press, pp 85–112.

TWO

Confidentiality, trust and truthfulness in professional relationships

Chris Clark

The problem

Professional codes of ethics standardly contain the expectation of confidentiality. The following plain and concise statements from the General Medical Council can well serve as a working definition of the principle as it applies in all the personal service professions (GMC, 2000):

> Doctors hold information about patients which is private and sensitive. This information must not be given to others unless the patient consents or you can justify the disclosure. (p 1)

> Patients have a right to expect that information about them will be held in confidence by their doctors. Confidentiality is central to trust between doctors and patients. Without assurances about confidentiality, patients may be reluctant to give doctors the information they need in order to provide good care. If you are asked to provide information about patients you should:

>> Seek patients' consent to disclosure of information wherever possible, whether or not you judge that patients can be identified from the disclosure.
>> Anonymise data where unidentifiable data will serve the purpose.
>> Keep disclosures to the minimum necessary.

> You must always be prepared to justify your decisions in
> accordance with this guidance. (p 2)

The familiar core principle of confidentiality is well elaborated in the
literature (for example, Beauchamp and Childress, 1994; Clark, 1995)
and its import will therefore be taken for granted in the following
discussion.

Professional codes also contain at least an implied expectation that
professionals will tell the truth. Typically this is much more indirectly
and less clearly expressed than the expectation of confidentiality. The
following are representative discussions of the expectation of honesty
or truth-telling.

From the field of medicine, Beauchamp and Childress (1994, p 307)
comment that: 'Surprisingly, codes of medical ethics generally ignore
rules of veracity', explaining the concept 'veracity, an obligation to
tell the truth and not to lie or deceive others'. They propose three
arguments for rules of veracity in relationships between healthcare
professionals and patients: that veracity is part of the respect we owe
others; that it follows from the obligation to keep promises; and that
it is necessary for fruitful interaction and cooperation. But they note
that 'nondisclosure, deception and lying will occasionally be justified
when veracity conflicts with other obligations' (p 309). Begley and
Blackwood (2000), for example, raise the issue that full disclosure of a
poor prognosis may harm the patient by destroying hope; Gold (2004)
points out that Western ideas of truth-telling may not always transfer
easily to multicultural contexts.

In social work, Clark (2000) identifies 'honesty and truthfulness' as
one of eight rules of ethical practice in social work. 'Social work services
should be offered and given in a manner that is honest, open, truthful
and transparent to users' (p 51). More than merely avoiding deception,
it requires positively striving to ensure the user's good understanding
of the service process.

Banks remarks that codes of ethics for a range of professions including
architects, engineers, health-related professions and social work generally
contain statements about the attributes of the professional, such as
'professional practitioners should be honest, trustworthy and reliable'
(Banks, 2004, p 109). From the professional associations, the code of
the (American) National Association of Social Workers (NASW, 1996)
declares that in pursuit of the value of integrity, '[s]ocial workers behave
in a trustworthy manner ... act honestly and responsibly'. Similarly, in its
Code of Ethics, the British Association of Social Workers (BASW, 2002)
declares that '[i]ntegrity comprises honesty, reliability, openness and

impartiality, and is an essential value in the practice of social work'. The British Association for Counselling and Psychotherapy (BACP, 2002, p 4; emphasis in original) likewise requires '**Integrity:** commitment to being moral in dealings with others, personal straightforwardness, honesty and coherence'.

From the domain of official regulation, the codes issued by the Scottish Social Services Council (2005, paras 2.1, 2.2) require that social service workers must 'strive to maintain the trust and confidence of service users and carers' by 'Being honest and trustworthy' and 'Communicating in an appropriate, open, accurate and straightforward way'.

I shall take it in this discussion that honesty means consistent and conscientious representation of the truth as one believes it to be, and the avoidance of intentional misrepresentation. It also means the avoidance of guile, deceit or misleading – the intentional creation of misunderstanding in the mind of the listener. As we have seen in the examples above, truthfulness in communications seems on first inspection to be the necessary counterpart of a disposition to honesty. I shall argue, however, that truthfulness is more complex than merely a commitment to actual veracity or accuracy. It is by way of a fuller exploration of the entailments of truthfulness – and its counterpart, trust – that we shall be better able to disentangle the apparently conflicting expectations of confidentiality as a principle of professional–client relationships.

The principles of confidentiality and truthfulness in professional relationships are, we are assured by the professional codes, designed to serve client interests. Examination shows, however, that the ends served by observing confidentiality and truthfulness respectively are liable to be in conflict. Let us consider in turn the client's interests in his (or her) direct relationship with the professional, and his interests that the professional is supposed to be pursuing on his behalf.

In his relation to the professional the client values confidentiality because it preserves his (or her) secrets and protects his privacy. In a professional working relationship guarded by confidentiality the client will feel more free to disclose his hopes and fears, faults and weaknesses, misdemeanours and errors. He will be able to discuss, as often he must, how his predicament and its resolution may impact on his family, relationships and whole way of life. Such disclosures will enable the professional to best help the client by opening the way to a fuller, clearer, shared understanding of the client's needs and expectations.

In his relation to the professional the client values the professional's truthfulness for reasons akin to those for confidentiality. He needs to trust that the professional will not deceive or mislead him. He will gain an accurate idea of what is and is not being done on his behalf, and the reasons for this. His trust in the professional will develop as it is based on his growing experience that what the professional says in the context of the helping relationship proves to be a good guide for addressing his problem.

If we compare this picture of the client's expectations of how the direct working relationship with the professional is served by confidentiality and truthfulness with how the client's interests are best served by the professional outwith his or her direct contact we find a dissonance. In order to best help the client the professional may choose to communicate information gained in confidence. The standard ethic of confidentiality says that such passing on of information must be sanctioned by the client's informed consent, that information passed on must be limited to what is minimally necessary for the work in hand, and that its disclosure must be limited to the smallest number of recipients necessary. But this is not how it works in practice (Clark, 2006). The client's confidential information is often very widely distributed without his full understanding, and including content that he supposed was to remain private. What is happening therefore is that the professional and the agency are transmitting information that the client naively imagines is to remain private, not out of negligence or malice, but in order to serve the client's interests: the infringement of confidentiality is thus justified by the professional's legitimate purposes.

There is a similar paradox in relation to truthfulness. In order best to pursue the resolution of the client's problem, the professional may quite deliberately choose to disclose less than the full truth to other parties in the situation. In part, of course, this is a direct consequence of striving to maintain such a degree of confidentiality as the case merits: as a professional I will refrain from disclosing a great deal of what I know about the client precisely in order to preserve confidentiality; but to do so I may have to resort to half-truths or pretence or evasion, with an obvious cost to whole truthfulness. Beyond that, as the client's agent or advocate the professional will very deliberately select aspects of the truth for presentation to other parties. Lawyers face the strongest version of this predicament because, in order to represent the client, they may be required to deliberately declare in public what they privately know to be untrue. Professionals in other contexts have to make the best case they can for the help and resources that the client needs, often in a context of scarcity and competition; they will choose what part of the truth to present; they will aim for the most favourable construction of the client's position in order to avoid social or legal sanction.

The problem for professional ethics can therefore be stated as follows. As regards confidentiality, professionals are simultaneously expected both to adhere to a strong version of it and selectively breach it for good professional reasons. As regards truthfulness, professionals are again simultaneously expected both to practise it in high degree and compromise it for the sake of other legitimate ends. We have what may be termed an *external* conflict in professional ethics between the *ends* served by confidentiality and truthfulness, respectively. This conflict is external in the sense that the ends of confidentiality and truthfulness are in part other-regarding. At the same time, of course, confidentiality and truthfulness are not independent expectations or standards because the practice of truthfulness relies on the shelter of confidentiality; and the practice of confidentiality is absurd unless it deals truthfully with the client's privacy and secrets. We have, then, what may be termed an *internal* conflict in professional ethics between the practices of confidentiality and truthfulness. This is an internal conflict because it poses issues of self-consistency in the pursuit of the values associated with confidentiality and truthfulness respectively.

Truth-telling and trust

Just like the professional codes, the ordinary precepts of common morality command honest talking and straight dealing. What is it that depends on the practice of truthfulness? And how shall we address the commonplace paradox that while accepted standards of morality universally discountenance lying, lies or half-truths of one sort or another seem to be both ubiquitous and indispensable in everyday social intercourse?

In 'Truthfulness, lies and moral philosophers' Alasdair MacIntyre (1995) suggests that there are three kinds of issue in the debate between those philosophers, including Mill, who regard some kinds of lying as permissible, and those, notably Kant, who regard the prohibition on lying as permitting no exception. The first is whether a lie is to be defined by an intention to deceive (by those in the first camp) or an intention to assert what is false (in the second). The second concerns the nature of the offence: whether it is a matter of the harm inflicted on social relationships and trust or whether a lie is to be deprecated because it calls into question the liar's standing as a rational person. The third set of issues concerns the justification of lies. Those who hold that some types of lie are permissible focus on the effects of lying, while the other camp is concerned with the nature of the act of lying. Thus, MacIntyre argues, one tradition regards lying primarily as an *offence against truth* – 'an error-engendering misuse of assertion' – while the other regards it as an *offence against credibility and trust* – 'having effects that tend to be destructive of relationships between persons' (MacIntyre, 1995, pp 316-17).

Working by a completely different route, in *Truth and Truthfulness* Bernard Williams (2002) develops a 'genealogy' of truthfulness in which, broadly, he argues that humans in society benefit from a division of the labour of gaining true and useful information about the world. This labour is advanced by dispositions to acquiring correct beliefs and to saying what one actually believes. So for Williams, Accuracy and Sincerity are 'the two basic *virtues of truth*' (Williams, 2002, p 44; emphasis in original). Summarising Williams, Elgin (2005, p 345) succinctly puts it in this way: 'Accuracy is the disposition to believe truths. Sincerity is the disposition to say what one believes'.

Taking a lead, then, from these two contemporary philosophers, we can say as a first approximation that truthfulness is to be valued for two main kinds of reasons. First, truthfulness promotes true knowledge and understanding of states of the world, including understanding of the content of others' minds. True knowledge – Williams' Accuracy – is indispensable to human flourishing; without it we cannot conceive of even a primitive or rudimentary human community relevantly distinguishable from the associations of animals. Second, truthfulness – Williams' Sincerity – is ordinarily necessary to sustaining relationships of trust, cooperation and mutual support. If we cannot believe that our fellows are speaking truly we cannot treat their statements as reliable indications of their beliefs or intentions, or as valid indicators of states of the world. And without relationships of cooperation and support, human life would be unbearable if not actually impossible.

The core of the problem for the practical ethics of honesty is thus that the argument for truthfulness seemingly stands on two separate and independent justifications, each having impressive face validity and supported by long and deep tradition in morality. The two bases of justification do not, however, necessarily lead to similar or compatible prescriptions for practical action. There are several potential strategies for addressing this issue. One might be to show that one or other of the two justifications is without moral or conceptual merit. Given the ubiquity and depth of the two principles, this does not seem a promising or plausible approach. A second approach would be to show that one was logically superior to the other – for example, that truth-telling should always take precedence over care for the feelings of one's fellows or the ill that might consequently befall them. This much-rehearsed argument, famously attributable to Kant, is discordant with the vast majority of contemporary opinion. A third approach is to show either that one principle is substantively reducible to the other, or that both are in fact derivatives of some higher principle, so that the conflict is only apparent. A fourth approach is to show that the contradictions are a result of faulty concepts and reasoning and can be resolved by more advanced analysis.

Whatever may be the merits or the potential of such theoretical strategies, in ordinary moral discourse none has secured the kind of universal support that would make it feasible or defensible, in the real world, to forget about either of the two principles of accuracy and sincerity. Since professionals have to work with the world as it actually is they must therefore deal with two principles that survive as functionally independent. And given two practically independent principles, the contrariness of the world can be relied on to throw up an endless series of situations where satisfying one involves infringing the other. For the practical ethics of honesty, both in professional life and elsewhere, we shall have to work on the assumption that both principles will need to be satisfied as best they may; and that we shall therefore need tools for prioritising the interests of sincerity and accuracy according to the demands of the occasion.

Truthfulness and trust in professional relationships

Truthfulness is apparently necessary to serve the essential principles of accuracy and sincerity in communication; but equally, accuracy and sincerity in real-life communications are liable in some circumstances to be damaged by an over-literal application of veracity, or plain unvarnished truth-telling, if that means something like 'the truth, the whole truth and nothing but the truth'. There is a whole host of reasons why one does not utter everything one knows that might conceivably be contextually relevant: because it would obscure more important and urgent communication; because time and opportunity are limited, and choices about what to say and what to omit are inevitable; because it would distract or mislead; because one does not wish to impose or coerce; because it would be needlessly threatening, frightening or offensive to the listener; because it would infringe the rights or interests of other parties. A great part of the socialisation of children involves learning what to say and what not to say according to the requirements of the context. The embarrassment caused when mistakes are made about the expectations of veracity is universally familiar, as is the repertoire of conversational devices that are deployed to repair relations after the fact.

Professionals necessarily work within the ordinary rules of conversation, and indeed may be faulted if their command of them is poor; every doctor who treats patients face to face needs a reassuring bedside manner as well as a knowledge of medicine. But professionals also work partly outside the rules of ordinary social interaction. They probe and challenge on matters, and in a manner, that would be intolerable outside the practice of their professional role; they require the confiding of information that would ordinarily be regarded as private and not for sharing with anyone other than a chosen intimate. In the client's contact with the professional the usual expectations of the limits of truth-telling may be radically challenged as the client must tell the professional about matters that would ordinarily remain private. The professional, too, is reciprocally bound by special rules about truth-telling, including the rule of confidentiality and the obligation to communicate some kinds of sensitive information even if the client is unwilling to sanction it. These mutual and complementary expectations of the professional relationship show that the requirement of truthfulness is not to be equated with simple veracity. Truthfulness in professional relationships must entail something more than accuracy – the 'disposition to believe truths' and sincerity – the 'disposition to say what one believes'.

In her examination of the basis of professional relationships Koehn (1994) focuses particularly on the trust that needs to be reposed in professionals by both their clients and society at large. Koehn considers, and rejects, the argument that the authority of professionals is justified by their special expertise. Also rejected is the argument that professionals' authority derives from a species of quasi-legal contract entered into between the client and the professional. Instead, Koehn proposes that the core of the relationship is a pledge. Thus:

> A professional is an agent who freely makes a public promise to serve persons (e.g. the sick) who are distinguished by a specific desire for a particular good (e.g. health) and who have come into the presence of the professional with or on the expectation that the professional will promote that particular good. (Koehn, 1994, p 59)

Unlike a contract, which must be explicitly accepted by both parties to be binding, the act of profession – that is to say, the public declaration of taking on the professional role – 'binds the speaker upon utterance' (Koehn, 1994, p 59). The pledge can only be meaningful if embedded in reciprocal trust; so trust between professional and client is fundamental to the role and authority of professionals.

The merit of Koehn's analysis of professionalism is that it avoids grounding authority in the expertise of professionals, which is now very widely regarded as suspect, or in the notion of a contract, which Koehn comprehensively shows is no accurate representation of the power relationships between professionals and clients. The argument that professional authority can be founded entirely on a pledge seems, however, too weak to either explain or legitimate the authority that is wielded by professionals employed by or on behalf of the state. Koehn's analysis is informed by a traditional and perhaps fictitious conception of the professional as a member of an independent guild governed by its own precepts and standards, and such a picture will plainly not cover the position of the large majority of health and social service workers who are in fact employed by the state or state-funded agencies. Despite this weakness, Koehn is surely correct to insist that the relationship between professional and client must be underpinned by trust. The good faith of the client must ultimately rest on the good intentions of the professional. Without the professional's sincere pledge of disinterested service, no amount of legal contract or official regulation will adequately protect the vital interests of the client.

We have seen that in relationships between clients and professionals honesty, sincerity, truthfulness and cognate virtues are expected as a matter of course. But truthfulness is complicated, and leads to expectations that conflict with each other. If we accept Koehn's argument that trust is paramount, we can find a way to resolve the paradox sketched above, that is, that despite the acknowledged good reasons for the general expectation of truth-telling in professional relationships there are, in ordinary social practice, innumerable good reasons for limiting the utterance of truth, or what I have termed simple veracity. In short, in the fabric of relationships trust is more important than mere truth-telling, so norms of truth-telling need to be modified by a different reading of truthfulness than simple veracity.

What are the expectations of truthfulness in the context where trust is the prior good? Trust requires fidelity to the nature of the relationship to take precedence over simple veracity merely for its own sake. In a relationship of trust I count on your telling me what will best fulfil the expectation of personal respect, or fellow citizenship, or friendship, or disinterested service, or love, which I take the relationship to be founded on; and I trust too that your expectations are shared and reciprocal to mine. Truthfulness in this context is cognisant of the many restrictions on what it is relationally beneficial to say and what it is practically possible to say. Truthfulness carries, and is sustained by, a certain unspoken, implicit knowingness about the arena of truth in which it is played out.

This conclusion has some affinities with MacIntyre's analysis of whether lying is ever justifiable. Although MacIntyre wants to defend a strong, almost Kantian, prohibition on lying, he finds nonetheless that on rare occasions it will be justifiable to lie in order to prevent a horrendous crime: his examples are the protector of a Jewish child against the Nazis, and the mother of a child threatened by a man bent on murder. Characteristically, he focuses on the social context of relationships and argues that instead of first asking, in Kantian fashion, "'By what principles am I, as a rational person, bound?'" we should first ask "'By what principles are we, as actually or potentially rational persons, bound in our relationships?'" (MacIntyre, 1995, p 352). MacIntyre proceeds to the conclusion:

> The rule we need is one designed to protect truthfulness in relationships.... 'Uphold truthfulness in all your actions by being unqualifiedly truthful in all your relationships and by lying to aggressors only in order to protect those truthful relationships against aggressors, and even then only when lying is the least harm that can afford an effective defense against aggression'.(MacIntyre, 1995, p 352)

My point of concurrence with MacIntyre is thus to conceive of truthfulness primarily as an attribute of *relationships* and to distinguish it from simple truth-telling or veracity as a feature of *statements*.

Truthfulness is, then, not best thought of as a species of moral commandment or deontological law; it is not identical to Sincerity, the disposition to say what one believes. Equally, truthfulness is not best thought of as an epistemological injunction; it is not the same as Accuracy, the disposition to believe truths. Truthfulness is rather a virtue to be cultivated by professionals, and others; and it is to be practised in the context of professional and other relationships. The practice of virtue does not admit the imposition of rigid abstract rules, but requires instead the exercise of flexible practical judgement, formed through experience, in the infinitely variable contexts of social life and daily decision making. To orient this daily intuitive decision making that is undertaken by all socially competent individuals we might think, in Aristotelian fashion, of truthfulness as a mean between two vices. On the one hand, we should avoid excessive veracity – too much information, albeit accurate information – of the wrong sort, in the wrong context, at the wrong moment, to the wrong listener. On the other hand, we should equally avoid dishonesty, whereby information (whether true or false) or implication is deployed with intent to deceive and disadvantage the listener. The touchstone of truthfulness is trust, and trust is a property of relationships.

For professionals the virtue of truthfulness will acquire a special character adapted to their professional role; the truthfulness required of professionals is different from the truthfulness expected of private citizens. The reasons for this are to be found in the non-symmetrical nature of professional–client relationships. The ordinary relationships of love, kinship, friendship and community depend on reciprocation of the transactions and trust between the parties. The reciprocation is usually imperfect, of course, and may well be marked by uncertainty and ambiguity. Nevertheless, it is universally understood by all competent social actors that such relationships are of *mutual* benefit. By contrast, the relationship of professional to client is avowedly for the prime benefit of the client and only incidentally for the benefit of the professional. Thus, it is a universal feature of professional codes of ethics that the client's interests must take precedence over the professional's.

The professional virtue of truthfulness, then, is moulded by the professional's pledge of service (as Koehn puts it) and the expectation that he (or she) will efface his own interest in favour of the client's. This may be imagined as a disposition to sincerity that is nevertheless ruled over by a kind of perpetual inner watchfulness – a watchfulness whose first concerns must always be the benefit of the client and the profession's wider obligations to the public good. Perhaps indeed this virtue of watchful truthfulness requires professionals, on occasion, to utter statements that must lie some substantial distance from Accuracy; perhaps as members of the wider community we intuitively and implicitly understand this, even if it is not widely admitted; perhaps this is a defining feature of professionalism itself.

Watchful truthfulness and its implications for professional confidentiality

For professionals, truthfulness is no literal and unmodulated truth-telling. Confidentiality, which guards the space in which truthfulness in professional relationships can flourish, is thus no simplistic rule of non-disclosure. What are the implications of the professional's moderated or watchful truthfulness for the practice of professional confidentiality? Social work and other publicly legitimated services are characterised by complex accountability (Clark, 2000, p 83). The professional's accountability is not merely to a solitary client, but to a number of individuals who are related to the client in a network of mutual expectations and obligations. Equally, the professional's accountability is not limited to the client and the client's kin, but extends in other, and sometimes conflicting, directions towards a wider accountability for the welfare of other members of society and the general public good. The professional virtue of truthfulness must therefore be moderated by the professional's multiple and complex accountability. Thus, the requirements of professional confidentiality can be analysed into obligations in three spheres: (i) directly to the client, (ii) to the rights and needs of proximate others, such as the client's kin and (iii) to the wider public good.

In the professional's direct relationship with the client, the simple precept of confidentiality as non-disclosure of personal information without prior explicit consent is moderated, as argued above, by a priority of truthfulness in the relationship over literal and undiscriminating veracity. For the sake of the integrity of the relationship it will occasionally be necessary to make disclosures that the client has not explicitly sanctioned. This occurs primarily when the client is judged to have less than full capacity or mental competence, whether through immaturity or mental or physical impairment. Hughes and Louw (2002, p 147), for example, argue that in dealing with patients with dementia 'confidentiality cannot be an overriding principle'; practice must necessarily focus on the social context in which patients with dementia are managed, and this requires sharing confidential information for the patient's good.

Despite the traditional concept of the professional and client voluntarily contracting to enter a closed dyadic relationship dedicated to the pursuit of the client's ends, professionals in health and social care do not deal with individuals in isolation from their social networks. As in other aspects of the relationship, the practice of confidentiality is moderated by a watchful truthfulness that must have regard for the rights and needs of proximate others. This follows directly from core principles of professional ethics including respecting persons and the protection of autonomy: the principle of respect is universal in its application, and cannot be applied preferentially to the identified client at the expense of other individuals in the client's life.

For similar reasons, therefore, and also by reference to the accepted grounds for the special rights and privileges of professionals, the practice of confidentiality is moderated by watchful truthfulness towards the wider public good. Thus it is that professionals should warn their clients that the expected standard of confidentiality of the client's disclosures is liable to be moderated or even entirely overthrown if it is judged necessary to protect vulnerable others or, as we might equally say, to maintain the expected standards of trust and truthfulness towards the wider public.

The relationship between professionals and clients starts out from a presumption of confidentiality, for familiar reasons well rehearsed in the lore and literature of the professions. Excavation of the grounds for this presumption reveals an indispensable concern for the rights and autonomy of users of professional services, together with a commitment to protecting truthfulness of communications between professionals and clients. This truthfulness is widely agreed to have both intrinsic and instrumental value. Truthfulness, however, is not a simple attribute or a straightforwardly defined virtue. Folded within it are what Williams (2002) pictures as Accuracy and Sincerity; and I have argued that, at least for the purposes of defining the requirements of professional relationships, Accuracy sometimes has to give way to Sincerity.

The obligation of professional confidentiality can thus be pictured as a three-cornered contest of the professional's truthfulness towards the individual client, towards others proximate to the client and towards the wider public good. Because excess fidelity to Accuracy towards one or other corner may well prejudice the proper interests of the others, I have characterised the professional's truthfulness as a watchful truthfulness, which must be ever mindful of how serving one good cause can easily bring about injury to another equally good one. While there can be no simple formula for balancing these interests, I have proposed that professionals should concentrate on cultivating a broader virtue of truthfulness that will equip them to make balanced judgements on the daily run of cases. This watchful truthfulness may, perhaps, be a more cautious, imperfect and compromising standard than moral theories often seem to countenance, but it seems to suit the case better than moral codes embracing lofty principles destined to be chronically ignored.

References

BACP (British Association for Counselling and Psychotherapy) (2002) *Ethical Framework for Good Practice in Counselling and Psychotherapy*, Lutterworth: BACP.

Banks, S. (2004) *Ethics, Accountability and the Social Professions*, Basingstoke: Palgrave.

BASW (British Association of Social Workers) (2002) *The Code of Ethics for Social Work*, Birmingham: BASW.

Beauchamp, T.L. and Childress, J.F. (1994) *Principles of Biomedical Ethics* (4th edition), New York: Oxford University Press.

Begley, A. and Blackwood, B. (2000) 'Truth–telling versus hope: a dilemma in practice', *International Journal of Nursing Practice*, vol 6, no 1, pp 26-31.

Clark, C. (1995) 'Competence and discipline in professional formation', *British Journal of Social Work*, vol 25, pp 563-80.

Clark, C. (2006) 'Against confidentiality? Privacy, safety and the public good in professional communications', *Journal of Social Work*, vol 6, no 2, pp 117-36.

Clark, C.L. (2000) *Social Work Ethics: Politics, Principles and Practice*, Basingstoke: Macmillan.

Elgin, C. Z. (2005) 'Williams on truthfulness', *The Philosophical Quarterly*, vol 55, no 219, p 343-52.

GMC (General Medical Council) (2000) *Confidentiality: Protecting and Providing Information*, London: GMC.

Gold, M. (2004) 'Is honesty always the best policy? Ethical aspects of truth telling', *Internal Medicine Journal*, vol 34, no 9-10, pp 578-80.

Hughes, J.C. and Louw, S.J. (2002) 'Confidentiality and cognitive impairment: professional and philosophical ethics', *Age and Ageing*, vol 31, no 2, pp 147-50.

Koehn, D. (1994) *The Ground of Professional Ethics*, London: Routledge.

MacIntyre, A. (1995) 'Truthfulness, lies and moral philosophers', in G.B. Peterson (ed) *The Tanner Lectures on Human Values*, Salt Lake City, UT: University of Utah Press, pp 309-61.

MacIntyre, A. and Dunne, J. (2002) 'Alasdair MacIntyre on education: in dialogue with Joseph Dunne', *Journal of Philosophy of Education*, vol 36, no 1, pp 1-19.

NASW (National Association of Social Workers) (1996) *Code of Ethics*, Washington, DC: NASW.

Scottish Social Services Council (2005) *Code of Practice for Social Service Workers and Employers*, Dundee: Scottish Social Services Council.

Williams, B. (2002) *Truth and Truthfulness: An Essay in Genealogy*, Princeton, NJ: Princeton University Press.

THREE

Confidentiality in practice: non-Western perspectives on privacy[1]

Ian Harper

Introduction

After being trained in medicine I worked as a doctor in hospital medicine and general practice in the UK. Since 1990 I have both worked in Nepal as a medical practitioner and researched into the practices of medicine and public health as an anthropologist. I have been responsible for recording patient data onto notes, their storage in remote clinics, and their transfer as part of trials of tuberculosis (TB) treatments and their outcomes in remote parts of Nepal. I have talked to patients and their relatives about their medical diagnoses in situations where health is frequently understood in quite different ways than the UK. I have carried out ethnographic studies in clinics and hospital spaces, interacting with patients and health workers, and interviewing policy makers and members of the community. In this chapter I draw on these diverse empirical experiences to reflect on the idea of 'confidentiality' both from an interdisciplinary perspective and in the non-Western context of Nepal. I pose questions about whether Western notions of privacy and confidentiality are ethnocentric, and the extent to which they can be applied elsewhere.

When we think of confidentiality there seems to be a lacuna in the literature, namely questions of cultural difference. I provide these examples of my experience as a tentative introduction of cultural difference into the debate. Despite there being wide differences in context, particularly in legal provision, consumer rights and the capacity of the state, I hope that these reflections on cultural difference, ethical relativism and the question of multidisciplinarity in Nepal's health field may also be of use for debate in multicultural Britain.

Medical treatment in Nepal: private space and public knowledge

Adjusting to Nepal for the first time can be difficult. One of the first things that anyone visiting has to get used to is the apparent lack of privacy. The notions of individual private space that we appreciate in the UK are challenged. This invasion of private space can be experienced as quite profound culture shock. The squeeze of the crowds; the kids staring in through the windows of your flat; the way that others can listen in to what we think of as personal conversations are a few of the numerous examples. That invisible social shield around us, experienced as an extension of our being and developed from our experiences at home, can feel threatened and violated. The reverse is true for Nepali friends who arrive in the UK: the emptiness of the streets; the lack of support, particularly of the family; the apparent lack of certain forms of sociality. Family support structures in Nepal extend way beyond the nuclear family to extensive networks distributed across the country. The cultural differences, experienced aesthetically, emotionally and physically, can be profoundly disorienting and disturbing.

Historically, anthropologists have even theorised the whole of South Asia as fundamentally different on the basis of those societies' relationship to individualism. Louis Dumont (1980) based his entire structural and holistic analysis of Indian society on its absolute opposition to 'Western' individualism. Other theorists have developed notions of Indian sociality as based not on individualism, but rather on the sense of self that those in South Asia develop from the 'dividual', who is inherently linked to others (Marriot and Inden, 1977). While these positions have been challenged as being ethnocentric and too sweeping, the point remains that forms of sociality and notions of the individual do appear significantly different.

There is a very wide range of healing practices in Nepal and throughout South Asia that are frequently based on entirely different epistemological and ontological principles, ranging from Ayurveda to the practices of shamans, mediums and herbalists. Nepal's extraordinary cultural and ethnic diversity makes for an eclectic range of healers, and there is little space here for discussion on the relationships between these healers, ethnic identity and their place in modernity and the functionings of the modern state. However, as we move from the family and the street into what might broadly be construed as healing spaces, what is striking is that healing rituals are largely performative and involve far more people than just the individual affected and the healer. The rituals of mediums and shamans, for example, as numerous monographs and writings on Nepal attest, always involve large numbers of the extended family and community members as the performances unfold. Whenever I have witnessed these sessions there is always a crowd gathered around listening, engaging and commenting on what is going on. The individual is not the only one being affected by these sessions, and some have argued that they are by no means the most important focus, since issues in the community are also articulated and resolved (via idioms of 'witchcraft', for example, or spirit possession).

When we move from these spaces to the medical clinics and hospitals this difference travels with us. Reissland and Burghart (1989) have shown how in maternity clinics, it is the extensive family support and local cultural values, and not the medical rules and determinations, that establish the forms of medical care. My visits to outpatients in Nepal have always been challenging in this way. For example, I was recently in the psychiatric outpatients department of a major hospital in Kathmandu. To my surprise, it was a very crowded small room, and there were two desks, each with two doctors at them, with the desks separated by a cupboard. This meant that there were four patients being seen by four doctors in a space where they could all be overheard. Histories were being taken to elicit personal data towards a mental health diagnosis; patients' relatives, friends and those of other patients stood by listening in to, and contributing to, the doctor–patient conversations as diagnoses were being arrived at and treatments dispensed. There was little sense of privacy here at all, and save for the generally obfuscatory language of medicine – new terms were applied, as the treatments were prescribed – these encounters were for all intents and purposes conducted in public space. This remains as difficult for me to accept today as when I myself practised medicine in East Nepal in the early 1990s. The expectation that the patient should be the first to be presented with confidential information was not how many health workers I worked with saw things; frequently it was the relatives who were informed first, or at least at the same time. A rejoinder to my sense of disquiet would be along the lines of this is not how we do things in Nepal, in short the evocation of a sense of cultural difference. Nonetheless, many of the worried ill with stigmatising conditions (such as TB or some forms of mental illness) will travel some distance to receive treatment out of sight of neighbours and community members.

In another hospital where I was researching in the TB clinic, staff were assisting in a survey by the National Tuberculosis Programme of HIV incidence among new smear-positive TB patients. This was part of the general sentinel surveillance system to monitor the levels of HIV in those with smear-positive TB. The trial had been set up so that the results would be anonymous and could not be traced to individual patients. However, the identification numbers for the trial were recorded in the patients' notes, so that when the results came back to the clinic, staff did see the results and knew who was infected with HIV. When they found out the individuals' results the staff asked me, how could they not then treat these patients and give them counselling? When I pointed out this anomaly to the medical director of the hospital, he said that they were aware of it, but the staff defended the practice by saying that in Nepal their culture is different (the idea of cultural relativism and patient disclosure I return to later). Disturbing for me was that those with HIV sitting in the outpatients department were generally known as such to the staff; on several occasions waiting patients were pointed out to me (in English – so they wouldn't understand). A general knowledge circulated among the staff and this in part seemed to be facilitated by the geography of the outpatients department. The cubicles were overcrowded and separated by curtains, so that it was easy for others to move in and out, and again the idea of personal space and private hospital space I had experienced in the UK was significantly challenged.

In a series of clinics set up for the treatment of TB in East Nepal in the early 1990s, the staff of the organisation were concerned with the links between TB and HIV. While the treatment of TB would not have been any different, it was felt that it would be useful for the staff to know the HIV status of the patient, so that we could then treat any other conditions that the patient might develop from this (this was prior to the advent of anti-retroviral drugs), and counselling could also be developed. There were, however, few services available at the time, and the associated social stigma was very strong. For example, the local papers took it upon themselves to release the name of a woman returned from Bombay who had developed AIDS. Her house was stoned and she was run out of town. We felt that, given the level of stigma and the total lack of any services at the time to support those with HIV, that it was best just to do what we did – treat the TB well. A similar situation occurred during my later research when a local paper published the names of some sex workers, and that they had been tested for HIV, resulting too in the women leaving the area. Such knowledge and rumour can circulate rapidly through dense informal and other networks with potentially devastating consequences.

Yet, apparently paradoxically, in many ways patients have greater control of their records and their personal data in Nepal than in the UK. Different issues tend to arise therefore around the sharing of patient data. I know of only a few hospitals in Nepal where data (or at least outpatient data) are kept on a central computerised database. Data gathering from records is rudimentary. In many institutions outpatients themselves are made responsible for carrying their notes and these are not kept in the hospital at all. I am still frequently asked to give advice to the unwell. They always have their notes, x-rays and blood reports with them – even if they don't understand what has been written on them. How different this is to my experience as a general practitioner (GP) in the UK, where we would wait weeks for the transfer of notes (this was before the computerisation of patient record keeping) and the control of patient data was firmly in the hands of the medical system (this has now changed with the Data Protection Acts, but still requires that patients know their rights).

In Nepal, however, the practice of patients keeping their own notes tends to compound a particular problem of continuity of treatment, especially for the chronically unwell. The tendency is to visit multiple practitioners, and the consequent overprescribing of medications is a particular problem. No one registers with a single GP in Nepal, as this system has never been developed; rather the tendency is to visit those doctors who have a reputation (via rumour, from friends, family and neighbours), frequently heading straight to tertiary treatment centres. Many people shop around for treatment from place to place, bringing their notes and being made responsible for them. In such circumstances the issue is not so much the release of personal data by the institution but rather the patients and their families circulating poorly understood notes, blood and other tests themselves as they seek help from multiple sites.

This raised a different ethical dilemma in those patients and in families I spoke to. During the course of my PhD fieldwork I encountered a case of a healing (Harper, 2003). A young man, a trained health worker who had visited a number of health institutions, had received ritual treatment from a *lama* (the local name for shamans – those who enter into a trance to divine the cause of a problem) and had been divined as having been cursed by a witch. The witch was being driven from him by a particular treatment whereby a hot ladle is applied to the body and if the shaman's divination is correct the witch is burnt and not the individual. This event was attended by many observers including over a dozen concerned family and friends. The following day the relatives brought me his medical notes to look at and asked if it could possibly be witchcraft, and whether it was alright to combine the 'medical line' and '*lama* lines' of treatment. His notes stated that he had been simultaneously treated for depression with fluoxetine, a fact of which he had been unaware; it was felt that the 'multiple physical complaints' he had experienced were indicative of depression. While he and the family had control of the notes, they were still largely unaware of their medical contents, yet remained happy for me to write this story in my field notes. My research into the emergence of psychiatric services indicated that patients were rarely told the diagnosis, in large part because of the associated stigma of being labelled as having a mental health problem.

I was then, and still am, asked to assess the treatments of the worried ill. They and their families will bring their notes with them. The notes are not always easy to decipher, but it is possible to discern the names of clinics, the diagnoses made and tests carried out, and the brand names of drugs prescribed. In discussion with these individuals, and in conjunction with my observation of the often very short consultation times they have with medical practitioners, it becomes apparent that they are frequently unsure of the rationale for treatments given. One young man, for example, came asking for advice after he had visited numerous clinics both in India and Nepal. His diagnostic profile ranged from malaria through to gastritis and he had been treated unsuccessfully for these conditions. After I travelled with him to a mission hospital he was eventually diagnosed with TB and placed on treatment. The question of disclosure here was firmly in his hands. Such disclosures tended to reveal the difficulties of interactions with health practitioners and institutions.

One final example from the implementation of the World Health Organization's (WHO) TB policy in Nepal provides further challenges to notions of confidentiality. I was particularly struck by the difficulty and struggles that the staff were having as they attempted to introduce new treatment protocols. The way the protocols were being implemented resulted in some patients being denied access into the programme (Harper, 2005, 2006). During the research I was asked to present a paper on the subject of local politics in the introduction of the TB policy at an international conference organised by the WHO in Kathmandu. As I discussed with the staff what I might present, I was asked by one key proponent responsible for the introduction of the programme not to disclose certain information I had gathered during the fieldwork. His concern was that it was better to keep certain things hidden from his superiors in the programme, and let them know what they wanted to hear, as he put it – namely that the programme was being correctly implemented and the protocols were being followed. In fact this was not happening, as a number of the health staff felt – wisely in my opinion – that the 'directly observed treatment' demanded by the protocols was unworkable. The key proponent was concerned that this would reflect poorly on him, and, worse, his position might be in jeopardy. There were widespread rumours and no few examples of how, in a very hierarchical system, those who upset their superiors could be transferred out to other districts, or lose training perks. The head of the National Tuberculosis Programme was also under considerable pressure within the competitive world of health development practices to demonstrate the success of the national programme.

Protecting the autonomy of the individual?

The ethical guidelines of the Association of Social Anthropologists (Association of Social Anthropologists, 1999), which most anthropological practitioners use to guide their practice, frame ethical issues as a series of responsibilities. Listed first is our responsibility for protecting our informants' interests. The practices I was researching in Nepal were also a subject of research commissioned by the National Tuberculosis Programme, funded by the Department for International Development and implemented by researchers from the Nuffield Institute in Leeds. This research was developed to feed into the development of national policy in relation to what form of direct observation was best for patients. The district I was in had been randomly selected for a trial and the female community health volunteers were being used for this purpose. As well as respect for the wishes of the health workers, what was also at issue was that their practices in relation to the introduction of the policy had broader implications for public health. This would apply not only in Nepal but also further afield because the results of this research would feed into international debates into what forms of observation are best for patients (see Newell et al, 2006). An argument from a consequentialist ethical position could equally be mustered to defend overriding the wishes of the project worker mentioned above.

Ethical debates in anthropology have recently focused on the question of informed consent for the use of qualitative ethnographic data. The debate on this tends to spin out from two general positions. On the one hand is a concern that with the iterative nature of anthropological participant observation research, researchers often do not know in advance what the outcomes will be. The difficulty with informed consent in these research contexts is that 'unlike the doctor who can give some, albeit limited, idea of the potential outcome of a procedure, an anthropologist cannot, and should not, hope to control the effects of his or her interactions' (Kelly, 2003, p 190). The counterpoint emphasises that there is no way out of the changing (Euro-American) context of increased regulation. As Fluehr-Lobban (2004, p 165) argues:

> A thematic concern with the protection of the individual and personal autonomy is apparent in the development of government regulation.... This protection of personal autonomy is, ultimately, the primary justification for informed consent provision, so the question that emerges is the degree to which this particular history applies to behavioural science and anthropological research and their practice. I would argue that it does so not only on moral and humanistic grounds, but also because anthropological and social science research is increasingly subject to the same.

A concern in the UK has been how the law and legal issues have come to dominate questions of anthropological ethics (Harper and Corsin-Jiminez, 2005). In short, these tend towards the legalistic; they anticipate legal consequences and assume a defensive idiom that can vitiate a full moral discussion of the issues. With regard to the medical realm more generally, the international standard now drawn on to guide medical practice and research is the Declaration of Helsinki. The four main issues this document highlights are: respect for the autonomy of the research participants; the risk of harm; the quality and value of the research; and justice (Hope, 2004). The focus on informed consent, like confidentiality, falls firmly in the arena of respect for the autonomy of individuals.

But in a similar vein to informed consent in international medical research, the question remains as to the degree that this protection of the autonomous individual's right to consent is an ethnocentric imposition. As has been noted in a heated debate in the US on ethics in anthropology following the publication of Tierney's (2000) *Darkness in El Dorado*, and the accusations in it that anthropologists were complicit in illegally conducted medical research, Hill argues that there are differences in the degree of consent required for the disclosure of information in experimentation, observational research and epidemiological surveillance. Consent is not necessary, for example, for routine epidemiological surveillance (Hill in Borofsky, 2005, p 185). Hill argues that in between experimentation and public health surveillance there is a wide range of public health research that may, or may not, be important for broader issues of well-being.

As well as there being different requirements of consent for the release of information according to the nature of the research, the other argument raised in anthropology is one of relativism. Again there is an oscillation between the position that respect for other cultures and beliefs requires informed consent and the contrary view that obtaining consent is ethnocentric as it depends on a particular idea of the individual; the latter can be used as an excuse for not getting informed consent (Fluehr-Lobban, 2004, p 171). The anthropological tendency to argue from a position of ethical and moral relativism is a slippery slope. There is a large gap between respect of difference, and the extreme position of suggesting that any cultural practices should be respected and tolerated equally (Macklin, 2006). However, applied judiciously, an understanding of cultural relativism is a useful heuristic device. In an anthropological intervention into ethical questions of medical research in the developing world, Parkin (2002) argued that an appreciation of cultural difference is important. He highlighted that the usual focus on individuals is an externally derived Western cultural view, which stresses notions of individual rights, over other locally defined possibilities, like paternalism. Looking at the question of agreeing to participate in research or not in a situation where certain individuals, particularly women, might not be culturally empowered to speak was a question of some considerable difficulty, and required sensitive subjective assessment (Parkin, 2002). The trouble is that it is easy to slip from a nuanced understanding of relativism into a position that justifies any number of potential abuses. When this relativism is applied to justifications for lower standards of care for participants in medical research than in richer countries, for example, the debate is heated; the counterargument is that such 'apologists' should not be tolerated and interpretive loopholes in ethical regulation need to be removed (Landes, 2005).

The question of context here is crucial to prevent these discussions from becoming too abstract and general. Anthropologists have long argued that in thinking of bioethical issues more attention needs to be paid to the lived moral worlds and experience of illness and suffering in specific contexts (Kleinman, 1995; Marshall and Koenig, 1996). With research this local context involves, crucially, attention to the poor and marginalised and their lived worlds. As Farmer and Campos (2006, p 256) point out, drawing on the debate that emanated from anti-retroviral studies in Uganda where volunteers were not offered treatment, institutional review boards are concerned more with the law, 'not pragmatic ethical engagement with the interests of the study subjects'.

Similar debates have played out in ethical discussions in the caring professions (Hugman, 2005); questions of the universal and the particular, of cultural difference, of the relationship between ethics as law and as guidance and the degree to which ethics oscillates between the individual and the social have surfaced in the development and implementation of ethical codes in the caring professions in Euro-American contexts. Shifting between these different positions Hugman is led towards a discussion of Habermas and 'discourse ethics', a position that focuses on process rather than specific principles (Hugman, 2005, pp 137-9). This, in theory at least, allows all those with a stake in the ethical process to have a say and be heard; those are the conditions under which dialogue about values and actions in professional practice should be conducted. It allows for the often competing theories and ideas (like the different positions a deontological and utilitarian ethics might allow in the Nepal examples I have given) to be played out in practice. This position assumes ideas of democracy and the communication this facilitates as primary. It cannot be taken for granted that this is what all the actors in the process value. Yet for the complex, multilayered investments in the question of disclosure of information I have described in Nepal this seems to me the best way forward, without prioritising any absolutist position.

Conclusion

I have briefly presented a range of contexts and issues that emerged from my work and research in the health field in Nepal, and how these impact on questions of confidentiality. In presenting ethical dilemmas such as these I find it impossible to take the moral or ethical high ground as to a particular course of action. My experience has led me to be suspicious towards the idea that there can be one universally applicable standard of confidentiality in health settings in a country like Nepal. The situations are complex and the ethical ambiguities faced in real-life situations of practice and research make appropriation of any particular position difficult and fraught with uncertainty. This is worth taking into account when we think of issues of globalisation, and the attempts that particular institutions might make in trying to push one particular form of ethical stricture developed elsewhere.

At the Association of Social Anthropologists we have suggested that rather than ethical guidelines being normative and regulatory, they should be developed for the purposes of education, as a means to think through the multiple, and frequently competing, ethical responsibilities that arise in research (Harper and Corsin-Jiminez, 2005). We have argued that more descriptive and ethnographic accounts and case studies are needed that emphasise the ambiguities and ethical dilemmas. In the

Nepal context, the question of confidentiality is complicated by the fact that the patients and their families already have control of their notes. The significance of this is less than clear when the diagnoses, and potential implications of these diagnoses, are poorly understood by those who hold them (and when indeed they are written in language the holders may not understand – that is, both in English and using medical terminology). In what ways do the apparent permeability of kinship and other networks impact when these continue in the hospital spaces and exchanges with doctors? How does this challenge the notions of individuality that we hold so dear, and suffuse our suggested ethical regulatory structures?

What might be the implications for multicultural Britain? I am not sure that sets of prescriptive solutions are the answer. As the UK is far more highly regulated than Nepal with respect to ethics and confidentiality there is inevitably going to be a greater degree of acquiescence to legal and professional norms. A starting point might be to place under question the discourses from which they arise and by which they are dominated – that is, the combination of medical expertise and legal sanction. As an anthropologist I would argue that we should attempt to understand the context (including the 'cultural' and political-economic context) of the interactions that constitute the development of normative rules around confidentiality. One issue might be to try to understand the complexity of relations around cultural ideas of the individual, family and cultural expectations of encounters with the health service. What are the issues at stake when members of a diaspora – like the ever-increasing numbers of the Nepali community in the UK – hold expectations and notions of the individual that differ from the normative framework of medicine and the law? Viewed from this perspective, and the rigorously experiential and empirical, we might begin to develop a picture of what is at stake.

Note

[1] Some aspects of this chapter, with a more specific focus on researching into Nepal's TB programme, appear in Harper, I. (2007) in a special edition of *Social Science and Medicine* on informed consent.

References

Association of Social Anthropologists of the UK and the Commonwealth (1999) *Ethical Guidelines for Good Research Practice*, www.theasa.org/ethics/ethics_guidelines.htm

Borofsky, R. (ed) (2005) *Yanomami: The Fierce Controversy and What We Can Learn From It*, Berkeley, CA: University of California.

Dumont, L. (1980) *Homo Hierarchicus: The Caste System and its Implications*, Chicago, IL: University of Chicago Press.

Farmer, P. and Campos, N. (2006) 'New malaise: bioethics and human rights in the global era', in B. Bennet (ed) *Health, Rights and Globalisation*, Aldershot: Ashgate, pp 255-63.

Fluehr-Lobban, C. (2004) 'Informed consent in anthropological research: we are not exempt', in C. Fluehr-Lobban (ed) *Ethics and the Profession of Anthropology: Dialogue for an Ethically Conscious Practice* (3rd edition), Walnut Creek, Lantham, NY: AltaMira Press, pp 159-77.

Harper, I. (2003) 'Magic, mission and medicalisation: an anthropological study of public health in contemporary Nepal', PhD thesis, University of London.

Harper, I. (2005) 'Interconnected and interinfected: DOTS and the stabilisation of the tuberculosis control programme in Nepal', in D. Mosse and D. Lewis (eds) *The Aid Effect: Ethnographies of Development and Neo-Liberal Reform*, London: Pluto, pp 126-49.

Harper, I. (2006) 'Anthropology, DOTS and understanding tuberculosis control in Nepal', *Journal of Biosocial Science*, vol 38, no 1, pp 57-67.

Harper, I. (2007) 'Translating ethics: Researching public health and medical practices in Nepal', *Social Science and Medicine*, vol 65, pp 2235-47.

Harper, I. and Corsin-Jiminez, A. (2005) 'Towards interactive professional ethics', *Anthropology Today*, vol 21, no 5, pp 10-12.

Hope, T. (2004) *Medical Ethics: A Very Short Introduction*, Oxford: Oxford University Press.

Hugman, R. (2005) *New Approaches in Ethics for the Caring Professions*, Basingstoke: Palgrave Macmillan.

Kelly, A. (2003) 'Research and the subject: the practice of informed consent', *PoLAR*, vol 26, no 2, pp 182-95.

Kleinman, A. (1995) *Writing at the Margin*, Berkeley, CA: University of California Press.

Landes, M. (2005) 'Can context justify an ethical double standard for clinical research in developing countries?', *Globalization and Health*, vol 1, no 11, http://globalizationandhealth.com/content/1/1/11

Macklin, R. (2006) 'Ethical relativism in a multicultural society', in B. Bennett (ed) *Health, Rights and Globalisation*, Aldershot: Ashgate, pp 153-74.

Marriott, M. and Inden, R. (1977) 'Towards an ethnosociology of South Asian caste systems', in K. David (ed) *The New Wind: Changing Identities in South Asia*, The Hague: Mouton, pp 227-38.

Marshall, P. and Koenig, B. (1996) 'Bioethics in anthropology: perspectives on culture, medicine, and morality', in T. Johnson and C. F. Sargent (eds) *Medical Anthropology: Contemporary Theory and Method* (2nd edition), New York: Praeger, pp 349-73.

Newell, J., Baral, S., Pande, S., Bam, D. S. and Malla, P. (2006) 'Family-member DOTS and community DOTS for tuberculosis control in Nepal: cluster-randomised controlled trial', *Lancet*, vol 367, pp 903-9.

Parkin, D. (2002) 'An anthropological experience of talking about medical research ethics', *Anthropology in Action*, vol 9, no 3, pp 6-41.

Reissland, R. and Burghart, R. (1989) 'Active patients: the integration of modern and traditional obstetric practices in Nepal', *Social Science of Medicine*, vol 29, no 1, pp 43-52.

Tierney, P. (2000) *Darkness in El Dorado: How Scientists and Journalists Devastated the Amazon*, New York: Norton.

FOUR

Ethical practice in joined-up working

Ian E. Thompson

An approach from practice

In this chapter the approach will be to work from the actual needs of practice to agreed ethical policy and procedures. Here we seek to follow Aristotle's advice to proceed a posteriori rather than a priori in our exploration of the issues involved in handling personal information. Aristotle argued that ethics is a practical science, intimately connected with law and politics, and that these form part of the same continuum – embracing in one frame the personal, communal and sociopolitical aspects of our sharing of power and responsibility in any moral community. Aristotle's approach is in a broad sense empirical and proceeds from practical experience towards the formulation of decision procedures and evaluative criteria. He emphasises the crucial role of 'prudence' in practical decision making, requiring not only knowledge of ethical principles, but also skills based on practical experience and the development of standard policies and rules through the exercise of actual public accountability (Thomson, 1976).

The focus in this chapter will be on the kind of policy and procedures that are needed to deal with issues of confidentiality and privacy in professional practice, and the practical requirements for responsible institutional management of personal information. I will examine and compare two cases where I have been directly involved as a research consultant. The first example is from Western Australia, where inadvertent disclosure of personal health information in the press provoked calls for the Minister of Health to resign and necessitated the development of policy and procedures to deal with the ensuing crisis. The second relates to developing a youth justice strategy within the Integrated Children's Services Plan for the Outer Hebrides. This task was undertaken in the context of intense media interest over the arrest of 13 adults and nine people charged with child abuse, followed by a surprising decision by the Crown not to proceed with the case. There were also local concerns over community safety, with an ageing population feeling threatened by the antisocial behaviour of a small group of young people.

The emphasis here will be on ethics as a practical discipline that requires training and the acquisition of skills in values clarification and ethical decision making; it needs to be based on practical experience rather than abstract moral theorising. Thus, to deal with issues of confidentiality and privacy in everyday practice requires standardised methods and tools to make objective needs and risks assessments and so provide a sound evidence base for effective risk management. The key practical problems may be the lack of relevant training for practitioners and managers in information management, and the lack of experience in operating systematic methods for data recording and analysis rather than ignorance of ethical standards (CJSWDC, 2004).

Confidentiality, privacy and practical ethics

There is a deep and unresolved tension in our society between the demand for secrecy to protect individual privacy and confidential personal information and the opposing demand for transparency and public accountability of professionals in the public health and social services. While there appears to be broad agreement that the key terms involved in this debate should be clarified – terms such as 'secrecy' and 'transparency', 'confidentiality' and 'responsible information sharing', 'the right to privacy' and 'the public interest' – there is little agreement about how this should be done. Based on my practical experience, and despite being a philosopher, I would argue that clarifying these concepts is not primarily a matter of formal definition, but rather of developing procedures that distinguish these terms operationally and that can be cashed out in terms of improved standards of practice and effective safeguards for vulnerable service users. Ethical policy and procedures need to be negotiated and agreed at local level by actively engaging all relevant stakeholder groups.

For practitioners in healthcare and social work it is not self-evident how confidentiality should operate in consulting relationships with service users. In the area of child protection it is ironic that practitioners' respect for family privacy and secrets can and has enabled abuse to continue unreported. Development of ethical policy, standards and operational rules for confidentiality in practice, or safeguards to prevent breaches, is a practical task that needs to be addressed in the workplace by direct involvement of stakeholders. Experience in business and banking, whose approaches to management are frequently recommended in the public sector, is that compliance with ethical policy and standards is not achieved by a top-down regulatory approach, but by engaging key stakeholders, including customers, in the process to ensure their 'ownership' of the outcomes (George and Weimerskirch, 1994, ch 1; Sternberg, 2000, chs 2 and 8).

The 20th century was remarkable for the fact that the dominant views of ethics in Europe and the English-speaking world were either a type of privatised and psychologised view of ethics and values, or a meta-ethical view that competence in ethics requires knowledge of and ability to decide between different ethical theories. The former type, emphasising the subjective nature of moral decisions, was exemplified by psychological hedonism, act utilitarianism, situationism and the emotivist theory of values. The latter approach presented a radical choice between utilitarian and duty-based ethical theories as alternative ways of justifying moral judgements, and sought to achieve greater objectivity respectively by appeal either to facts or to unconditional moral imperatives. Utilitarianism has tended to relativise all ethical judgements as simply reflecting different interpretations of the facts about means and ends. Duty-based or deontological ethics has encouraged either a legalistic formalism or the 'tyranny of principles' (Jonsen and Toulmin, 1988).

From a moral-theoretic perspective, policies on confidentiality and privacy tend to be justified by one or more of the following theoretical positions:

- *principlism* – by appeal to the *deontological* principles of beneficence (or duty of care) and duty to respect personal autonomy (and 'right to privacy') (Bok, 1982; Beauchamp and Childress, 1994);
- *contractual* – by appeal to the implied or explicitly negotiated *rights and duties* of both parties arising out of care agreements with service providers (Thompson et al, 2006);
- *utilitarian* – by arguing that maintaining the trust and confidence of the service user is an essential *means to achieve the end* of effective intervention, or alternatively that personal confidences can be breached in the public interest (Singer, 1993);
- *virtue-based* – arguing for development of the *skills and dispositions* that engender service users' confidence in the security of their personal secrets (Hursthouse, 1999).

Siegler has gone so far as to argue that confidentiality in medicine is a 'decrepit concept', because of the increasingly complex, fragmented and corporatised nature of medicine and moves towards globalisation of healthcare and information systems (Siegler, 1982). In childcare the emergence of integrated children's services for the prevention of antisocial behaviour, child protection and reduction of youth crime mean that sharing of information between health, education and social services is increasingly necessary, both in the UK and within the European Community. While confidentiality may not necessarily be a 'decrepit concept' there certainly is a need for a more practical and grounded approach. The standard paradigm of confidentiality is challenged by growing awareness of service users' rights to be consulted about what personal information ought to be treated with strict confidentiality in the context of different cultural and legal assumptions about personal autonomy and community interests (Kerridge et al, p 128f). It is increasingly accepted that users have rights of access to their confidential records in making complaints, as practitioners have parallel rights to defend themselves against alleged negligence or misconduct when the information is relevant to litigation (CHIC, 2003). Information sharing for purposes of service planning, monitoring, evaluation of outcomes, performance appraisal, general research and service improvement (CJSWDC, 2004) also challenges confidentiality.

The systematically ambiguous nature of 'confidentiality' and the mystification of service users' 'rights to privacy' or 'rights to confidentiality' have tended to put these concepts beyond the scope of critical examination. It will be argued here that confidentiality and privacy are not principles in the sense of being logically primitive ethical concepts, but rather that they are operational duties derived from the more fundamental principles of justice, beneficence and respect for persons. This means that we need to shift attention from mere forms of words to the practical criteria required to appraise these operational responsibilities. Their scope will change in relation to the different contexts in which practitioners work, whether in one-to-one consultation, in teamwork, in institutional settings, or in interagency collaboration. The context will determine too how service users' personal information is managed, used and shared to plan and deal with service needs.

Moreover, while academics and administrators may be concerned with high-level general ethical policy and its justification, operational managers and practitioners are more concerned with how to apply ethical policy and general principles to actual cases and situations. There is an important distinction to be drawn here between case-based decision making and corporate decisions about higher-order policy principles. Moral decisions relate to specific situations, particular problems or dilemmas. Policies seek to formulate general rules to deal with recurring problems or situations. The responsibility and accountability applicable to the two levels are quite different and require different kinds of justification. In justifying general rules or ethical policies, we appeal either to higher authority, the law and law-givers, or to higher-level ethical theories. On the other hand, in justifying specific ethical or practical decisions it generally suffices to explain factually the nature of the problem addressed, what principles or rules we applied and with what caveats, what our objectives were and what means we chose to achieve our ends. It would not be appropriate or required of us, in court or at an inquiry, to engage in moral-theoretic discussion of the relative merits of different kinds of ethical theory.

Recently there has been a revival of a practical and experientially grounded ethics owing a debt to Aristotle. The rediscovery of virtue ethics, with its emphasis on the development of individual moral competencies and the need to build moral communities based on acceptance of the reciprocal relationship between rights and duties (Macintyre, 1981), has led to competency-based education and training for ethics in professional life (Thompson et al, 2006).

In practice, whether by instinct or training, we tend to apply the general steps in problem solving and decision making that Aristotle (Thomson, 1976) identified in characterising the virtue of prudence – the set of acquired skills required for making competent decisions. He argued that all ethical decisions are practical, directed towards problem solving, and are prudential in the sense that they must be informed by knowledge of the facts of the case and of relevant principles and rules, and will entail determining clear objectives and identifying the means available to achieve the best possible outcome.

It is my experience that the mystification of ethics has tended to obstruct the development of more practical forms of professional ethics relevant to everyday practice in modern urban and industrialised societies. Specifically, the common conflation of 'confidentiality' and 'privacy' would appear to rest on a tendency to overemphasise either the subjective nature of ethical principles or the theoretical nature of the issues involved. Mystification has also encouraged the view that education or skills training in ethics is unnecessary, because people are assumed to have some kind of direct intuition of what 'ethics' means. The challenge, however, is to *clarify the different kinds of rules and procedures that should be applied* in dealing with practical issues of privacy and confidentiality in different contexts (Windt et al, 1989, p 184f).

Law and policy

Recent developments in law have called into question the seemingly sacrosanct principles of confidentiality and the assumed right of health professionals to interpret its meaning in healthcare and the social services. No longer is it acceptable either to argue that confidentiality is some kind of unconditional imperative, because there are specified conditions under which it is our moral duty not to disclose information, or to argue in a professional context that decisions on whether to disclose information are simply matters of personal conscience. Instead, the law demands clear procedural arrangements for information sharing and practical methods for testing compliance or breaches (Kerridge et al, 1998, p 128ff; City of Edinburgh, 2002). For example, in 1976, in *Tarasoff v Regents of the University of California*, the California Supreme Court ruled that the clinical psychologist, Dr Moore, was negligent in *not* disclosing to Tatiana Tarasoff that his patient Prosenjit Poddor was threatening to kill her, which he subsequently did. In a landmark hearing in 1996 the New South Wales Supreme Court ruled in the case of *AM Strelec v D Nelson & 2 Ors* that Dr Nelson, a specialist obstetrician, had been negligent in not having kept adequate records of events that occurred in the course of his patient's labour. In 1996, in *Breen v Williams* (1996) 186 CLR 71, the issue of 'ownership' of medical records was decided by the High Court of Australia in favour of the originator of the record, and not the patient or service user, as tended to be argued by some under data protection legislation.

These and other cases have begun to form a body of case law that is redefining the scope and limits of confidentiality and the right to privacy. They have also sent shockwaves through healthcare systems worldwide, because there are now precedents for professionals being prosecuted or sued for failure to disclose information that puts others at risk, or for failure to keep adequate and systematic records – just as they previously risked court action for breaches of confidentiality.

Since the enactment in the UK of the 1998 Data Protection Act, the 2000 Freedom of Information Act and the 2002 Freedom of Information (Scotland) Act, there have been a number of publications giving procedural guidance on issues of privacy and breaches of confidentiality (DCA, 2002, 2003; PIU, 2002). Of particular relevance here are the findings of the national audit and review of child protection practice in Scotland (Scottish Executive, 2002), which highlighted the problems facing agencies and professionals in getting the right information at the right time to enable them to protect and support vulnerable children. The report insisted that information should be shared promptly with other agencies where children are at risk of abuse or neglect. The Scottish Executive's (2003) *Sharing Information about Children at Risk: A Guide to Good Practice* sought to clarify the legal position about confidential personal records and the circumstances under which sharing of information was not only permissible but mandatory, and set out practical guidance on procedures for sharing of information and suggested a format for the type of interagency protocols required. Its advice in summary was:

> If there is reasonable concern that a child may be at risk of harm this will always override a professional or agency requirement to keep information confidential. All professionals and service providers have a responsibility to act to make sure that a child whose safety or welfare may be at risk is protected from harm. They should always tell parents this. (Scottish Executive, 2003, p 3)

Failures to share information between practitioners or agencies, and/ or to compare available records and use them intelligently to inform critical decisions, have been repeatedly offered as serious criticisms in official reports on child abuse or youth crime. A notable example is *It's Everyone's Job to Make Sure I'm Alright* (Scottish Executive, 2002). Most such reports over the past quarter century have emphasised the critical need for improved information sharing and more 'joined-up' services, for example the reports of the Victoria Climbié and Caleb Ness inquiries (Laming, 2003; O'Brien, 2003; see also the recommendations in DH, 2000; Scottish Executive, 2000, 2002, 2006). However, integration and even co-location of different services does not necessarily improve information sharing, as was shown in the Caleb Ness inquiry (O'Brien, 2003). Practitioners from different agencies or services remain suspicious of one another and defensive of their own records. Reports have emphasised the need for training of staff in social services, healthcare, education, the police, housing and the independent sector in rigorous methods of child-centred assessment, information management and information sharing. New legislation in England and Scotland to deal with antisocial behaviour highlighted problems with interagency information sharing, which were partly due to the very different value bases and priorities of social work and health practitioners and the contrasting emphasis of the police and housing authorities on community safety.

In the 2003-04 Scottish Executive-funded Youth Justice Evaluation Project, the authors found that issues of the 'privacy' and 'confidentiality' of 'their' records were often used by practitioners and managers to justify not moving towards more joined-up service delivery. These findings were based on over 200 in-depth interviews and focus groups with youth justice practitioners and managers (CJSWDC, 2004). Respondents reflected defensive attitudes to sharing information with practitioners in other services or between agencies, and managers' attitudes reflected the same kind of institutional resistance, perpetuated by insular organisational cultures. Respondents argued against the introduction of more systematic methods of information management and transparent information sharing. They justified this because of conflicts of values with other services, and the sacrosanct privacy of 'their' service users' confidences. Managers also claimed proprietorial rights over 'their' records. It became apparent that managers did not trust their colleagues in other services to use sensitive information about service users appropriately. Alternatively, they appeared apprehensive that their record-keeping systems and information management would be shown to be deficient, or less than satisfactory when compared with those of other agencies. It became apparent that some changes in the law were necessary and that agreed national guidelines for practice in sharing information between different agencies needed to be developed. However, the research team also recommended that locally agreed procedures and interagency protocols for information sharing should be developed (CJSWDC, 2004).

The handling of sensitive personal information in cases where children are at risk, for example, requires practitioners who are well practised in responsible decision making and who keep good records of their decisions. For this to be possible and a matter of routine, requires good systems, effective management of services, and agreed procedures and protocols for the practical handling of information – so that decisions are not made arbitrarily or ad hoc. Practitioners must engage in critical self-examination and in personal and interagency values clarification if consensus is to be achieved on how and when it is appropriate for information to be shared. However, most critical decisions in areas of child protection or youth justice are not made by individuals on their own, but in consultation with their colleagues on the team or in case conferences where a group of practitioners from different professions may be involved. Recent Scottish guidance on standards has emphasised the need to respect the right of service users to be involved in action planning that affects them and decisions about their records being shared with other agencies, and that their views must be recorded (Scottish Executive, 2004; compare United Nations, 1989).

Perhaps of first importance is that records taken and kept must satisfy the practical principles of data protection (enshrined in the UK 1998 Data Protection Act). These duties are clearly set out in the National Treatment Agency for Substance Misuse's guidance on data protection and record retention (NHS/NTA, 2003), namely that data must be:

- fairly and lawfully processed;
- processed for limited purposes;
- adequate, relevant and not excessive;
- accurate;
- not kept for longer than is necessary;
- processed in line with the data subject's rights;
- secure;
- not transferred to countries outside the European Union without adequate protection.

The principles applicable to confidential relationships have long been established in common law and the courts have found a duty of confidence to exist where:

- a contract provides for information to be kept confidential;
- there is a special relationship between parties, such as patient and doctor, solicitor and client, teacher and pupil;
- an agency or government department, such as Her Majesty's Revenue & Customs, collects and holds personal information for the purposes of its functions.

However, no agency can guarantee absolute confidentiality as both statute and common law accept that information can be shared in some circumstances. Disclosure can be justified (DCA, 2003; Scottish Executive, 2003):

- if the information is not confidential in nature;
- if the person to whom the duty is owed has expressly or implicitly authorised the disclosure;
- if there is an overriding public interest in disclosure, for example a child or vulnerable adult is at risk;
- if disclosure is required by a court order or other legal obligation.

To make sound prudential judgements in difficult cases requires that we determine precisely: what information is confidential, whether service user consent has been given or can be legitimately assumed (for example in cases of mental incapacity), whether or not there is an overriding public interest, and whether the information will be required in the interests of justice. It is in relation to such matters that practitioners and managers need clearer organisational policies, procedures and support mechanisms to assist them to face difficult dilemmas and reach responsible decisions that they can justify publicly.

For example, practitioners and managers, in disclosing sensitive personal information need to be able to answer the following questions and to defend their answers in court if necessary (Scottish Executive, 2002; NHS/NTA, 2003):

- What is the purpose of the disclosure?
- What is the specific nature and extent of the information to be disclosed?
- To whom is the disclosure to be made (and is the recipient under a strict duty to treat the material as confidential)?
- Has the service user been consulted about the proposed disclosure of his (or her) records?
- Is the proposed disclosure a proportionate response to the need to protect the welfare of the service user, for example a child, to whom the confidential information relates?

Ethical policy development in practice – two case studies

The approach I advocate in this chapter can be justified on theoretical and philosophical grounds, as I have attempted to do so far, but it can perhaps be more convincingly demonstrated on the basis of my practical experience and the research in which I have been engaged with colleagues. Two practical examples will be discussed – the first from Australia and the second from Scotland. The first involved the remit to review existing policy and develop a strategic plan and practical procedures for the handling of confidential health information in the state of Western Australia (CHIC, 2003). The second was concerned more indirectly with rights of privacy and issues of confidentiality in the context of strategic and operational planning for child protection and youth justice in the Outer Hebrides (CJSWDC, 2004; CnES, 2006).

In both these cases it became apparent that there was a lot of confusion among practitioners and managers about the nature and scope of the rights of service users to confidentiality, the duties of those managing their personal information and confidential records, and the question of the 'ownership' of these records in the context of data protection and freedom of information legislation. As researchers we experienced defensiveness and resistance to the introduction of more rigorous and standardised forms of assessment, evidence-based practice and performance appraisal. This was mainly based on scepticism either that applying these methods would lead to service improvement or that sharing information would lead to better results or outcomes for clients. Respondents also appeared to feel that their autonomy as practitioners was under threat and in some cases appealed to the strict confidentiality of 'their' records to resist greater transparency and sharing of information with colleagues, or between agencies. What was significant in these two projects was the way in which many of these conflicts were resolved and consensus achieved by a process in which there was extensive participation of all key stakeholders in the interviews, focus groups and developmental workshops held.

Policy for handling confidential health information in Western Australia

In Western Australia an action research approach was adopted to develop a strategic plan and procedural guidelines for the handling of confidential health information throughout the State. The plan and guidelines were to meet both administrative needs and critical pressure from service users about the use of their medical records. The methods of investigation and policy development comprised semi-structured interviews, focus groups and service development workshops with all the identified stakeholder groups, including consumer and special interest groups, primary care and hospital physicians, administrators of medical records, information technology experts, social science and public health researchers, epidemiologists, and Health Department bureaucrats and health planners.

The project involved investigation of local needs and existing practice, including current methods for handling patient records in primary care and hospital settings. Matters investigated included how access to name-identified research data was scrutinised and approved for the purposes of evaluation of clinical treatment, for epidemiological and public health research, for health service planning, and audit; and procedures for dealing with complaints and litigation. Further, an examination was made of how individual projects were monitored and outcomes evaluated – the primary objective being to develop recommendations for the reform of existing practice endorsed by stakeholders.

The chief outcomes of the process in Western Australia were agreed policies and practical procedures for the handling of sensitive personal health information, and the formulation of strategic and operational plans for their implementation. Three years later these have not only been implemented but have been positively evaluated. Some examples of these agreed policies and practical procedures are shown in Box 4.1.

Box 4.1: Policies and procedures adopted in Western Australia

Procedural definitions to clarify the distinctions between: confidentiality and privacy; personal medical records and name-identified statistical data collections: 'identified', 'de-identified' and 're-identifiable' data, in line with national standards and local legislation.

Agreed quality assurance arrangements, including agreed terms of reference for the Confidential Health Information Committee (CHIC), standards for security of information storage, and procedures for examination and approval of applications for access to confidential information and monitoring of use made of information by applicants. A requirement for periodic external audit of the committee's work was also specified.

Agreed administrative arrangements and budget for staffing, information technology, data storage, management of the State's information resources and education of the public on their rights to confidentiality and freedom of information, and accessible information on the application process, review procedures, monitoring arrangements, networking of information between different agencies and methods for lodging complaints and appeals

Agreed forms for documents required, including copies of the code of practice for use of name-identified data from health statistical data collections, standard application forms, letters of approval, interagency information sharing protocols, final outcomes reports and termination declarations, and performance monitoring reports.

Agreed programme of staff and organisational development and funding to support it, to ensure that those responsible for the system were knowledgeable, skilled and competent to ensure its effective and efficient operation.

Other concerns identified by stakeholders were outwith the scope of the project (CHIC, 2003). These included the proliferation of organisations holding databases of personal information about people, including information of importance to their physical, mental or social well-being. Stakeholders were concerned about the rapid development and increasing power of information technology, in terms of the sheer volume of information about people that can be stored, exchanged and cross-linked, and the increasing potential for interlinking of databases, locally and nationally, without the explicit understanding or consent of the persons to whom the information relates. Other issues were the globalisation of healthcare systems and service provision, with the need for rapid international sharing of information and perhaps personal health information; and the need for international exchange of intelligence for the purposes of combating terrorism and drug and people trafficking.

Confidentiality and privacy in youth justice in the Outer Hebrides

The remit of the second project was to assist the local authority to conduct a youth crime audit and service mapping exercise using action research methods (similar to those used in Western Australia) in order to develop a strategic plan and operational procedures to help improve local services for young people. The aim was to reduce the risk of young people offending and to improve child protection and community safety (CnES, 2006).

Of direct relevance to this process was a concurrent high-profile official 'review, examination and investigation of the care and protection of children in Eilean Siar' by the Social Work Inspection Agency (SWIA). The review arose out of a situation where 13 adults were arrested on allegations of child abuse, nine being subsequently charged, and the controversial decision by the Crown not to proceed with the case. The SWIA (2005) report commended local practitioners for their thorough record keeping in this case and their sharing of information with other agencies. However, key practitioners were criticised for their lack of skill in the analysis and interpretation of available records in the light of research evidence, and for failure to use this knowledge to inform their decision making, resulting in delay in taking the children into care.

This case illustrates several important points in relation to the collection, sharing and use of personal information. First, efficient data collection does not mean that staff will be competent in the selection, aggregation and analysis of significant data; second, professional judgement based on personal experience is not enough, but must be informed by knowledge of the relevant research; and third, sharing of information between agencies needs to be as full and complete as possible, especially where children are at risk.

The delay and then failure of the English authorities to give full details of their records to Eilean Siar was criticised because it left the latter unaware of the extent of previous concern about the risk of abuse of the children by their mother's new partner, who had been previously convicted of child sexual abuse. The Health Board was criticised for its handling of health visitor records (which were either lost or destroyed) resulting in the team being ignorant of vital evidence of abuse. As a result, SWIA recommended adoption of a standard form of assessment across all agencies dealing with children in Scotland, and for the mandatory development of integrated Children's Services Plans by each local authority (SWIA, 2005).

In the face of the extensive local and national media coverage of the issues of child protection in the Western Isles, developing a youth justice strategy with local stakeholders proved to be a challenging process as people were initially very guarded and reluctant to be forthcoming in interviews and were suspicious of the motivation for the research. However, concern about the local case of child abuse helped to concentrate the minds of people on the need to develop an integrated approach to child protection, youth crime and community safety. This was partly because existing networks made good information sharing possible, albeit on an informal and ad hoc basis. Good local intelligence, in a close community, meant that key practitioners were well aware that essentially the same group of problem young people were the focus of concern in relation to child protection, youth crime and community safety. Paradoxically, while the priority given to youth crime by the Scottish Executive appeared to distort the emphasis in children's services, in reality it acted as a catalyst for better integration with initiatives on child protection and community safety. The process of conducting the youth crime audit, mapping of services for young people and developing the strategic plan took place separately at the start, but it resulted in better collaboration by all key agencies in the process of strategic planning for joined-up services and provided a model for improved formal sharing of information between local agencies.

Significantly, the Youth Justice Strategic Plan set out the agreements reached by senior representatives of the local Youth Justice Partnership to achieve better 'joined-up' services, based on well-supervised and accountable sharing of information. While concerns had repeatedly been raised about confidentiality, especially with the controversial child protection case in mind, it became apparent that in order to develop better child protection and youth justice services what was needed was an agreed information management policy, mutually agreed interagency policy, procedures and information sharing protocols.

Youth justice practitioners were intensively trained in the use of ASSET (a formal instrument for assessing the needs and risk of offending of young people) (Youth Justice Board, 2003) and progress was made towards regular collection, collation and aggregation of results. Similarly, the Western Isles Child Protection Committee developed practical interagency procedures and guidelines to deal with issues of child protection (CnES 2005).

Implications for service improvement

Twenty-five years ago Moore-Kirkland and Irey (see Windt et al, 1989, p 184f) argued that confidentiality in social work needed fundamental reappraisal, because current individualistic views of confidentiality were misleading and inappropriate when applied to the social contexts and working environments in which social workers operate. They stressed that social workers do not function as independent consulting professionals but exercise their roles within social systems circumscribed by law and regulation, and they have to intervene in the context of complex systems of relationships involving interactions with a variety of people, between a variety of statutory and other agencies. As they argued, confidentiality has become a portmanteau concept that needs to be unpacked – with different operational rules developed for its application in individual professional–client interactions, to team settings and management, and to organisational and interagency relationships. Skills in relevant forms of information management are required in each of these contexts, and ability to distinguish the operational rules that apply.

Against the background of reports on the Victoria Climbié case in England (Laming, 2003) and the Caleb Ness case in Scotland (O'Brien, 2003), there has been a reiteration by governments in both England and Scotland of the urgency of more effective 'joined-up services' to deal with child protection and youth crime (DH, 2000; Scottish Executive, 2005a, 2005b). For example, in the implementation plan for *Getting It Right For Every Child* (Scottish Executive, 2006), there is insistence on the need to develop: a single standardised assessment tool for children; competency-based training for frontline staff in assessment, data collection and analysis; and an improvement of practice in evidence-based action planning, monitoring and review.

A good model of an interagency information sharing protocol was jointly developed and piloted by The City of Edinburgh Housing Department and Lothian and Borders Police, as part of the wider Youth Justice Evaluation Project, while the work described above was going on in Eilean Siar. This contained five parts:

- *information* – explaining the law and the need for formal agreements and procedures for sharing information to prevent crime and antisocial behaviour and giving useful examples from both the housing and police perspectives;
- *explanations* – of the formal agreements, specific procedures in each agency to deal with requests for disclosure, and methods required to monitor that the use made of information shared between the different agencies is in accordance with the terms of the approval granted;
- *designated officers* – identifying a senior officer responsible for processing requests or initiating requests for information, and for determining the urgency of the request;
- *application form* – identifying the subject and his details, the legal or other grounds for the request, details of allegations against the subject, other relevant information;
- *notes of guidance* to practitioners on completing the form, and *advice* on where to seek professional or legal advice.

What is becoming increasingly obvious is that dealing effectively and appropriately with sensitive personal information, particularly about children's needs and risks, requires both practitioner skills and service systems that are fit for purpose, strategically and effectively managed. Developing fully integrated and strategically planned children's services demands the ability to correlate and compare vital intelligence about vulnerable children and families. This cannot be achieved without introducing sound evidence-based practice and systems of performance management, monitoring and appraisal.

However, introducing these cannot be achieved simply by prescription. Two decades of effort in the UK to introduce evidence-based practice and performance management in the National Health Service (NHS) shows that these efforts did not succeed until there was sufficient investment in staff and organisational development and direct involvement of stakeholder groups in the process (Muir-Gray, 2001; Harrison, 2004). This is also borne out by the evidence from business management where introduction of better systems of management and governance, such as the methods of total quality management (George and Weimerskirch, 1994; James, 1996), only works effectively when a fully consultative approach is adopted. This involves working directly with all key stakeholders in the specific organisation (and its partner agencies), through a recognised process, to develop relevant policy and procedures that they will collectively 'own', implement and adhere to in practice. In this way it becomes possible to 'cash out' the abstract principles in practical ways of working with service users, colleagues and other agencies that meet both ethical and legal requirements. On the basis of these collective, negotiated agreements and performance standards, the whole organisation, practitioners and management can be held publicly accountable and their performance measured (James, 1996).

From my experience of working with large organisations in ethical policy development and introducing performance management and evidence-based practice, I would argue that while much can be learned from examples of good practice elsewhere, issues around 'privacy' and 'confidentiality' cannot be effectively addressed without working with local employees at all levels to develop practical solutions and standards relevant to their needs. As research and practical experience of total quality management has shown, when it is applied as a holistic and values-driven process, in a genuinely consultative manner that involves all key stakeholders, then real benefits flow from the process. These are summarised in Box 4.2.

Box 4.2: Benefits of consultative methods for addressing issues of information management within and between organisations

- Agreed internal and interagency systems, procedures and protocols for the management and sharing of confidential records.
- Policy and procedures for supervision and monitoring, accountability in the management of personal information, and for research and evaluation.
- Conflicts within the service and with partners are recognised and can be dealt with.
- Enhanced competence in applied ethics, based on learning by doing.
- Identification of education and training needs.
- Improved teamwork and a real moral community among participants; mutual support to allay anxieties and subversion of change by denial.

- Modelling of meaningful forms of transparency and accountability; daily demonstration of the reciprocal relationship of rights and duties in practice.
- Preventing buckpassing because people accept responsibility for their roles and a duty of evidence-based accountability for their practice.
- Insight into how to improve organisational culture and public sector management.
- Helping to identify strengths in the organisation, and opportunities to build on achievements to develop good systems and procedures.
- Helping to identify weaknesses, and developing strategies to deal with faults. (compare DHSS, 1988)

References

Beauchamp, T.L. and Childress, J.F. (1994) *Principles of Biomedical Ethics* (4th edition), Oxford: Oxford University Press.

Bok, S. (1982) *Secrets: On the Ethics of Concealment and Revelation*, New York: Pantheon Books.

City of Edinburgh (2002) *Joint Protocol and Procedures for Sharing Information for the Prevention of Crime and Disorder*, Edinburgh: City of Edinburgh Council Housing Department and Lothian and Borders Police.

CHIC (Confidential Health Information Committee) (2003) *Strategic Plan for the Health Department of Western Australia on the Handling of Confidential Health Information*, Perth, WA: Health Department of Western Australia.

CJSWDC (Criminal Justice Social Work Development Centre) (2004) *Final Report on the Youth Justice Evaluation Project*, Edinburgh: The University of Edinburgh, Criminal Justice Social Work Development Centre for Scotland, (www.cjsw.ac.uk).

CnES (Comhairle nan Eilean Siar) (2005) *Inter-Agency Procedures and Guidelines* (July 2004 and July 2005 drafts), Stornoway: Western Isles Child Protection Committee.

CnES (2006) *Youth Justice Strategic Plan for Eilean Siar*, Stornoway: Western Isles Council.

DCA (Department for Constitutional Affairs) (2002) *Public Sector Data Sharing – Guide to the Law*, London: HMSO.

DCA (2003) *Public Sector Data Sharing – A Guide to Data Sharing Protocols*, London: HMSO.

DH (Department of Health) (2000) *Framework for the Assessment of Children in Need and their Families*, London: HMSO.

DHSS (Department of Health and Social Security) (1988) *Working Together: A Guide to Arrangements for Inter-Agency Cooperation for the Protection of Children from Abuse*, London: HMSO.

George, S. and Weimerskirch, A. (1994) *Total Quality Management*, The Portable MBA Series, New York: John Wiley.

Harrison, M.I. (2004) *Implementing Change in Health Systems: Market Reforms in the United Kingdom, Sweden, and the Netherlands*, London: Sage Publications.

Hursthouse, R. (1999) *On Virtue Ethics*, Oxford: Oxford University Press.

James, P. (1996) *Total Quality Management*, London and New York: Prentice Hall.

Jonsen, A.R. and Toulmin, S. (1988) *The Abuse of Casuistry: A History of Moral Reasoning*, Berkeley, CA: University of California Press.

Kerridge, I., Lowe, M. and McPhee, J. (1998) *Ethics and Law for the Health Professions*, Katoomba, NSW, Australia: Social Science Press.

Laming, Lord (2003) *The Victoria Climbié Inquiry*, Cm 5730, London: The Stationery Office.

Macintyre, A. (1981) *After Virtue* (2nd edition), Indiana: Notre Dame University Press.

Muir-Gray, J.A. (2001) *Evidence-Based Healthcare: How to Make Health Policy and Management Decisions*, Edinburgh: Churchill Livingstone.

NHS/NTA (National Health Service/National Treatment Agency for Substance Misuse) (2003) *Developing Drug Service Policies: Data Protection and Record Retention*, London: National Treatment Agency for Substance Misuse.

O'Brien, S. (2003) *Report of the Caleb Ness Inquiry*, Edinburgh: Edinburgh City Council.

PIU (Performance and Innovation Unit) (2002) *Privacy and Data Sharing*, Milton Keynes: Open University.

Scottish Executive (2000) *Protecting Children: A Shared Responsibility. Guidance for Health Professionals*, Edinburgh: Scottish Executive.

Scottish Executive (2002) *It's Everyone's Job to Make Sure I'm Alright – Report of a National Audit and Review of Child Protection Practice*, Edinburgh: Scottish Executive.

Scottish Executive (2003) *Sharing Information about Children at Risk: A Guide to Good Practice*, Edinburgh: Scottish Executive.

Scottish Executive (2004) *Protecting Children and Young People: Framework for Standards*, Edinburgh: Scottish Executive.

Scottish Executive (2005a) *Protecting Children and Young People: Child Protection Committees*, Edinburgh: Scottish Executive.

Scottish Executive (GIRFEC) (2005b) *Getting It Right For Every Child: Proposals for Action*, Edinburgh: The Stationery Office, www.scotland. gov.uk/publications

Scottish Executive (GIRFEC) (2006) *Getting It Right For Every Child: Implementation Plan*, Edinburgh: Scottish Executive, www.scotland. gov.uk/publications

Siegler, M. (1982) 'Confidentiality in medicine – a decrepit concept', *New England Journal of Medicine*, vol 307, pp 1518-21.

Singer, P. (1993) *Practical Ethics*, Cambridge: Cambridge University Press.

Sternberg, E. (2000) *Just Business: Business Ethics in Action* (2nd edition), London: Warner Books.

SWIA (Social Work Inspection Agency) (2005) *An Inspection into the Care and Protection of Children in Eilean Siar*, Edinburgh: SWIA.

Thompson, I.E., Melia, K.M., Boyd, K.M. and Horsburgh, D. (2006) *Nursing Ethics* (5th edition), Edinburgh and London: Elsevier.

Thomson, J.A.K. (tr) (1976) 'Nicomachean ethics Bk VI', in *The Ethics of Aristotle* (revised edition), Harmondsworth: Penguin.

United Nations (1989) *United Nations Convention on the Rights of the Child*, Geneva: United Nations.

Windt, P.Y., Appleby, P.C., Battin, M., Francis, L. and Landesman, B. (eds) (1989) *Ethical Issues in the Professions*, Englewood Cliffs, NJ: Prentice Hall.

Youth Justice Board (2003) *ASSET: Young Offender Assessment Profile,* Oxford: University of Oxford, Centre for Criminological Research.

Part Two
Balancing individual privacy with the right to information

The right to privacy and confidentiality for children: the law and current challenges

Lilian Edwards and Rowena Rodrigues

Introduction

How far should the law protect privacy? What balance should be struck between the individual's right to privacy and the interests of society? Should the privacy of the family bow to the duty on the state to safeguard the interests of vulnerable children and adults within a family? Should parents have the right to know everything about their children, or do children too need rights to a private sphere?

Questions like these have long been contested both in law and in society, and will recur throughout this book. They will not be solved in this brief chapter. Instead, we will consider the legal rules that seek to protect the privacy and confidence rights of individuals, focusing from time to time on how these rules operate for children and young persons. We will also consider some recent developments that illustrate how digitisation and the 'database society' are affecting privacy rights for children.

The two most important legal regimes to consider in privacy protection are data protection law, and the law of confidence. Data protection law in the UK has, since the 1998 Data Protection Act, been derived from a European Directive (outlined later) and thus exists in roughly harmonised form across the European Union (EU). The law of confidence, on the other hand, is a creature of the common law, and is idiosyncratic to English law (although Scottish law shares most of the same rules). Both regimes have been informed, and, in the case of the law of confidence, almost transformed in recent years, by the guarantees of a human right to a private life. This right is derived from the European Convention of Human Rights (ECHR), Article 8, especially since the incorporation of this instrument into UK domestic law in the 1998 Human Rights Act. Since the 1998 Act, the right to a private life as a fundamental human right can now be pled in any court in the land, with no need to go to the European Court of Human Rights in Strasbourg to raise the issue. Public bodies, such as local authorities and their social services and health services, must act in accordance with it and (in theory at least) legislation cannot be passed that breaches the ECHR.

Data protection law protects what is known very generally as *informational privacy*: the right to control what is known about you. The type of information protected is differently defined in different countries and is not always clear but typically includes 'personal data' such as name, address, date of birth, contact details, financial, medical and social work details, history of psychiatric treatment, photographs, genetic, racial and ethnic details, school records, domestic situation and so forth.

The law of confidence, by contrast, prevents a second party from disclosing information which should be kept private between that person and the one who revealed it. Historically, the law of confidence arose only in special well-known relationships of trust (for example between doctor and patient) or in a commercial 'trade secrets' context; however, as we shall see later, it is now evolving into the nearest thing the legal systems of the UK have to a general law of 'privacy'.

Privacy may, of course, also involve *physical* or bodily privacy – the right not to be touched or in some way acted on against your will. This area of law is grey in the extreme in the UK in its interaction with laws protecting autonomy, and may be dealt with under existing laws such as the criminal law of assault or rape.

Data protection

The coming of the information society and the impact on data protection

Informational privacy as a concept has its origins in the aftermath of the Second World War, Nazism and Stalinism. The pressing fear in Western states as the world rebuilt itself in the 1940s and 1950s was of the 'Big Brother state' that had been glimpsed in Germany and the totalitarian Soviet bloc. Data protection legislation thus began in states like Germany and Austria after 1945 and was first created as a harmonised European regime by the Council of Europe Convention of 1981.[1] It has since been adopted as mandatory law in the EU in the shape of the EC Data Protection Directive.[2] Rooted in the ECHR guarantee of a human right to private life in Article 8, data protection law was always intended to protect the privacy of individual citizens, and therefore, with some small exceptions, protects neither the deceased nor juristic persons (companies and similar unincorporated associations). It does, however, clearly protect children as well as adults.

At the international legal level, a range of instruments – including, for example, the Universal Declaration of Human Rights (UDHR, Article 12),[3] the International Covenant on Civil and Political Rights (ICCPR, Article 17)[4] and the European Convention on Human Rights (ECHR, Article 8) – all enshrine the right to private life and have all contributed to the creation of modern data protection law (Bygrave, 2002, p 116).

In the 1940s and 1950s, collection and processing of personal information by the state was achieved via conventional methods, such as census information gathering, internal passports, bureaucratic organisation and filing of paper data, and human surveillance. From the 1970s onwards, however, a new factor emerged: the arrival of the modern digital computer. The rise to prominence of data protection law in recent times is generally attributed to the increasing use of computers and electronic communication devices, with consequent privacy compromises and breaches (Carey, 2004, p 1). Works such as *Database Nation* (Garfinkel, 2001) and *The Unwanted Gaze* (Rosen, 2001) have publicised the idea that by virtue of information technology and ubiquitous electronic surveillance we are now living in a 'surveillance society' (Wood, 2006, para 11.3.3).

Computerisation and digitisation allow collection, processing and storage of personal data on a scale unprecedented in the analogue era. Huge amounts of data can be stored forever for relatively low cost, be searchable in minutes or seconds, not hours, by a vast number of criteria, and be processed in limitless numbers of useful ways. Crucially, data collected from one source or database can be combined with other databases, to generate new data revealing significant connections and comparisons.

'Profiling' – looking for patterns in the data collected or aggregated about a person or group of persons – has become ubiquitous. It is theoretically possible, for example, to combine someone's social security record with his (or her) employment and tax records at the touch of a button, generating correlations that might have serious privacy implications. In relation to groups of people, data, especially data combined from multiple databases, can be analysed statistically to produce predictions as to how persons in that group might behave in the future as a matter of probabilities and pattern recognition – the concept of 'data mining'. It might be predicted, for example, that a child from a certain postcode, school and social class of family might be more likely to become involved with social services or the police, than a child from a different data-profile background. Such predictions are, of course, not always correct, being merely based on probabilities, and decisions made relying on such data may be misguided or positively harmful. This is one of the major current controversies in relation to child information databases, and the rights of children to confidentiality and privacy.

Information held in databases for indefinite periods may also be reused for functions quite different from the purposes for which it was originally collected: this is the concept of 'function creep'. Data collected about a child for psychiatric counselling purposes, for example, might theoretically later be used to categorise the child as a risk in terms of law enforcement – something that the child could not have anticipated when data were shared and consent originally given. Data protection law tries to combat this by introducing restrictions, both on how long data may be retained and, crucially, on 'fishing' – collecting data for no particular purpose, or extremely wide purposes, and using such data as and when desired. Given the technical scope of modern computer storage and database technology, and the flimsy enforcement of data protection in practice (ICO, 2006a), however, such 'scope creep' may in practice be almost impossible to control. Indeed, Bennett and Raab (2006) suggest that it is one of the key hallmarks of the modern bureaucratic society that information *will* be collected just because it can be, as a valuable potential commodity for the unknown future. Such trends are worrying both for privacy activists and for today's children, who will have to grow up with the weight of already collected data metaphorically hung round their neck.

In current data protection law, the primary protection for the data subject is supposed to be the requirement that consent be obtained before personal data are disclosed or used. However, recent research by the Foundation for Information Policy Research (FIPR) (Anderson et al, 2006) has shown that both the law and the practice around *child* consent in the context of sharing of data about children, and law enforcement, are problematical. This is discussed later in relation to the ContactPoint child database soon to be created under the 2004 Children Act in England.

A further problematic aspect of digitised data processing is the non-transparency of decision making. As a result, data protection law includes the right of data subjects to see what data are held about them, and to correct errors. Decisions made wholly by automated means may always be challenged. In a child protection context, this means that a decision based solely on 'invisible' reasoning emerging from searches on large databases or combined databases may also be challenged.

The information society has, of course, now been transformed by the advent of the Internet. Our digital world has become ubiquitously connected and global. The Internet provides both ease of access to data by multiple data processors and instant transmission of data across the globe. This can be both empowering and concerning from a data privacy perspective. Since different laws govern rights of privacy and confidentiality in different countries, export and import of personal data may involve loss or gain of privacy rights. How to deal with the impact of different jurisdictions on data protection rights remains an opaque and politically thorny issue (Busch, 2006).

A final introductory issue about computerisation of data handling, especially in the interconnected Internet age, is data security. It is reasonably obvious if data held in handwritten files have been amended, or if the physical data store has been broken into; such interference is less obvious when data live on a hard disk. As a result, data security has also become part of the framework of data protection law.

Under the 1998 Data Protection Act, data controllers owe the duty to data subjects to protect the personal data they hold from accidental loss or dissemination and from third party hacking.

In November 2007, however, a severe blow was struck to the confidence of the UK public in the security of public sector databases when it was revealed that the details of some 25 million people including 7.25 million families – almost half the population of the UK – had been lost in transit when placed in an insecure postal service, on two unencrypted CDs, by a junior employee at Her Majesty's Revenue & Customs (HMRC). The two disks contained the names, addresses, dates of birth and bank account details of people who received Child Benefit; they also included National Insurance numbers. A swift inquiry, the Poynter Inquiry (HM Treasury, 2007), followed, as well as embarrassing revelations of many other public sector lapses in security in relation to personal data, by bodies ranging from the Ministry of Defence to the Driver and Vehicle Licensing Agency. The government publicly admitted that the loss of the HMRC Child Benefit data 'has raised questions about the safety of large-scale personal data in other government systems, including ContactPoint' (BBC News, 2007) and decided to postpone the rollout of ContactPoint by at least five months (see note 26). Not only is the security of the database now being questioned, but whether it is needed at all. Maria Miller, the Conservative shadow children's minister, commented: 'The government should also use this opportunity to see whether it really is necessary to have a database for every single child in the country, accessible to 330,000 people, given the significant amount of concern that this could overload the system and lead to a dumbing down of information' (BBC News, 2007).

Many commentators believe that the HMRC debacle may see the reversal of the UK's movement towards a 'database nation' (see page 100), which had earlier seemed unstoppable. The Information Commissioner is currently seeking drastically enhanced powers to audit, investigate and prevent data loss and data protection breach in general, including custodial sentences for those who breach the 1998 Data Protection Act. The EU Article 29 Data Protection Working Party, which supervises the operation of the Data Protection Directive (DPD),[5] also issued an opinion specifically on the protection of children's personal data in February 2008.

In March 2008, the influential Joint Committee on Human Rights, a UK parliamentary body, concluded that the HMRC data loss and similar incidents had resulted from '[a] fundamental problem ... there is insufficient respect for the right to respect for personal data in the public sector' (JCHR, 2008, para 27, p 14). Fixing this is likely to require a wholesale transformation of attitudes towards data protection compliance in both the private and public sectors. The JCHR has suggested that in future all statutes should be drafted to incorporate data protection principles, and that the general approach of drafting very wide enabling powers in primary legislation – such as section 12 of the 2004 Children Act – under which particular rules can be made by delegated legislation with very little scrutiny – should be abandoned. At the very least, it is likely that the public will take a far less trusting attitude towards the integrity, accuracy and security of public-sector and joined-up databases in the future, and that additional security safeguards will be required. What effects all this will have on the welfare of the children whose details were to be contained in ContactPoint (and other child-related public databases) remains to be seen.

Key legislative instruments: international level

The Data Protection Directive

The DPD is perhaps the most comprehensive and significant enactment on data protection in the world and was a positive step towards the harmonisation of data protection laws of member states of the EU. Adopted in October 1995, it was required to be given effect by national legislation in all member states of the EU by 24 October 1998. The UK passed the Data Protection Act (DPA) in 1998, which wholly replaced the earlier 1984 Act. The DPD has been extended to deal with technology challenges by the Privacy and Electronic Communications Directive 2002/58/EC, as implemented in the UK by Regulations in October 2003. This Directive aims at protecting the fundamental rights and freedoms of individuals, particularly their right to privacy. It aims to make sure that, in cases of flows of personal data between member states of the EU, the fundamental rights of individuals must be protected.

The substance of the DPD can be found in Article 6, which lays out the basic principles that must be followed in data processing except in cases where permitted exclusions apply. Article 6 states that member states shall provide that personal data must be:

(a) processed fairly and lawfully;

(b) collected for *specified, explicit and legitimate purposes* and not further processed in a way incompatible with those purposes. Further processing of data for historical, statistical or scientific purposes shall not be considered as incompatible provided that member states provide appropriate safeguards;

(c) *adequate, relevant and not excessive* in relation to the purposes for which they are collected and/or further processed;

(d) *accurate* and, where necessary, kept up to date; every reasonable step must be taken to ensure that data which are inaccurate or incomplete, having regard to the purposes for which they were collected or for which they are further processed, are erased or rectified;

(e) *kept* in a form that permits identification of data subjects for *no longer than is necessary for the purposes for which the data were collected* or for which they are further processed. Member states shall lay down appropriate safeguards for personal data stored for longer periods for historical, statistical or scientific use.

The DPD also sets out a number of conditions, at least one of which must apply, before personal data may be processed (Article 7). The most important justifying condition is that of consent, and what constitutes consent (see page 95). The DPD also bans the processing of personal data that reveals *sensitive personal data*, such as racial or ethnic origin, political opinions, religious or philosophical beliefs, trade union membership, offences, convictions, and health or sex life, unless such processing is justified[6] by one of its provisions (Article 8). In most cases, processing of sensitive personal data requires not just consent, which might be implied from circumstances or repeat behaviour, but *explicit consent*. Clearly, much data associated with child protection work will be sensitive personal data and fall into its more restrictive legal regime of protection.

Other key provisions of the DPD include:

(a) The data subject's fundamental right of *access to personal data* without constraint at reasonable intervals and without excessive delay or expense (Article 12(a)). Any person in theory is entitled to find out what data are held about them on a database. The right of subject access is, however, subject to a large number of exceptions, little used and is not in principle a right to prevent processing of that data (although see (c) below).

(b) The data subject's right to control the *integrity* of data relating to them, including the right to rectification, erasure or blocking of data whose processing does not comply with its provisions, in particular due to its incomplete or inaccurate nature (Article 12(b));

(c) The data subject's right to object (Article 14) in the cases listed in Article 7(e) and (f) at any time on compelling legitimate grounds to the processing of data (Article 14(a)), particularly where processing is *likely to cause damage or distress*, and in cases where personal data are used for direct marketing purposes (Article 14(b)).

(d) Article 15 provides that member states shall grant the right to every person not to be subject to a decision that produces legal effects concerning them or significantly affects them, based *solely on the automated processing of data*.

(e) Provisions for the *security* of processing of data are laid down in Article 17. These envisage the implementation and adoption of appropriate technical and organisational measures to protect personal data against accidental or unlawful destruction or accidental loss, alteration, unauthorised disclosure or access and so on.

The transfer of personal data to third countries is now provided for in Chapter IV of the Directive. Article 25 states that transfers of personal data to third countries may take place *only* if the third country in question also ensures an *adequate* level of protection, the adequacy of which would be assessed in the light of all the circumstances surrounding a data transfer operation or set of data transfer operations (Article 25(2)).

National level

The 1998 Data Protection Act

The UK 1998 Data Protection Act (1998 DPA) came into force on 1 March 2000, giving effect to the DPD. The UK system is policed by the Information Commissioner's Office (ICO), a body independent of both the government and commercial interests. A similar body exists in every EU state signatory to the DPD. Because of its independence, the ICO is, however, hampered both by lack of resources to fulfil its wide remit, and by lack of powers sufficient to deal with widespread flouting and ignorance of data protection law. The Information Commissioner has issued extensive legal guidance on the interpretation of the 1998 DPA and the principles and related issues (ICO, undated (a, b)). Data protection is a UK-wide matter reserved to Westminster. However, a Scottish Information Commissioner also exists, who has a role in relation to Scottish data protection interests as well as policing the Scottish Freedom of Information (FOI) scheme.

The 1998 DPA, like the DPD, uses certain specific and important terminology, most of which is defined in section 1(1) of the Act and is paraphrased here:

- **Data** means information that is being processed by means of equipment operating automatically, *or* is recorded with the intent that it should be processed by this equipment, *or* is recorded as a part of a relevant manual filing system.[7]
- **Data controller** is the person or company who *determines the purpose and manner* of the data processing. Most duties in the 1998 DPA are placed on data controllers.
- **Data processor** is the person who processes the data *on behalf of* the data controller, for example a data warehouse. Data processors in this technical sense are relatively unimportant in the DPA scheme.
- **Data subject** is the living person who is the subject of the personal data.
- **Personal data** are data that relate to a living individual who can be identified from those data, or with other data likely to be held by a data controller. The definition of personal data in the UK was significantly limited by the case of *Durant v FSA*.[8] In that case, the court held that:

> Mere mention of the data subject in a document held by a data controller does not necessarily amount to his personal data.

Whether it does so in any particular instance depends on where it falls in a 'continuum of relevance or proximity' to the data subject as distinct, say, from transactions or matters in which he may have been involved to a greater or lesser degree.

This definition has proved controversial and may yet be challenged in the European Court of Justice. In the context of children, it might conceivably be highly restrictive – for example, in a social work report compiled on child A, it is possible that a brief mention of information about child B, A's sibling, might not be regarded *ab initio* as personal data, thus restricting B's rights of access to those data, as well as other data protection rights.

- **Processing** is very widely defined to include obtaining, recording or holding the information or data on the data subject, or carrying out any set of operations on the data, *including* organising, adapting, altering, retrieving, combining, consulting, using, disclosing, transmitting or disseminating the data. It also covers blocking, erasing and destroying information or data.[9]

Part I of Schedule 1 of the 1998 DPA incorporates the eight data protection principles in the DPD (outlined earlier). Interpretative provisions that expand on the First, Second, Fourth, Sixth, Seventh and Eighth Principles are set out in Part II of Schedule 1.

The eight data protection principles as implemented into UK law can be summarised as follows:

(1) Personal data shall be processed fairly and lawfully.

(2) Personal data shall be obtained only for one or more specified and lawful purposes, and shall not be further processed in any manner incompatible with that purpose or those purposes.

(3) Personal data shall be adequate, relevant and not excessive in relation to the purpose or purposes for which they are processed.

(4) Personal data shall be accurate and, where necessary, kept up to date.

(5) Personal data processed for any purpose or purposes shall not be kept for longer than is necessary for that purpose or those purposes.

(6) Personal data shall be processed in accordance with the rights of data subjects under this Act.

(7) Appropriate technical and organisational measures shall be taken against unauthorised or unlawful processing of personal data and

against accidental loss or destruction of, or damage to, personal data.

(8) Personal data shall not be transferred to a country or territory outside the European Economic Area, unless that country or territory ensures an adequate level of protection of the rights and freedoms of data subjects in relation to the processing of personal data.

Fair processing as incorporated into the First Data Protection Principle is a crucial notion in giving teeth to rights of privacy for data subjects, especially for those seen as having more limited autonomy, such as children. The principal ground for rendering processing 'fair' is that the data subject has given his (or her) consent (DPD, Article 7; 1998 DPA, Schedule 2). Other grounds do exist, however, which will be of consequence in the context of social work and law enforcement: for example, that the processing is necessary to fulfil a legal obligation of the data controller (1998 DPA, Schedule 2, para 3), or that it is necessary to protect the data subject's 'vital interests' (1998 DPA, Schedule 2, para 4). The latter would be invoked, for example, if it was necessary to look at a person's medical records without his consent if he arrived in hospital unconscious. Consent may also not be necessary in certain cases where processing is undertaken in pursuit of statutory duties or under statutory powers.

Consent, oddly, remains undefined in the UK within the 1998 DPA. Within the DPD, Article 2, it is defined as 'any freely given specific and informed indication of his wishes by which the data subject signifies his agreement to personal data relating to him being processed'. This definition was not transposed into UK law on the supposition that the nature of consent was well understood in law. The ICO has indicated in guidance (ICO, undated (a)) that consent should be 'informed' and 'unambiguous'. The DPD definition of 'ordinary' consent should also be contrasted as something implicitly less rigorous than the (sometimes equally uncertain) requirement for 'explicit consent' for the processing of sensitive data, which is implemented in UK law (1998 DPA, Schedule 3, para 1).

Clearly, consent to the processing of 'ordinary' data can be *implicit* – that is, drawn from facts and circumstances or actions. Consent can also be *'opt-out'* rather than *'opt-in'* – in other words, a person can legally be asked as a form of consent to 'tick here if you do not wish your personal data to be shared with third parties' (a formulation often seen on consumer websites). The vagueness of the requirement of consent is one of the most problematic parts of modern data protection law. In many situations, consent will be given without anything resembling 'freely given specific and informed indication of [the data subject's] wishes' – for example, many standard form employment contracts require employees to consent to employer surveillance of their workplace, their emails and their telephone calls from work. Few employees will actually read and understand such clauses, and even fewer will turn a job down rather than give consent, there being effectively no possibility of negotiating on such standard terms.

When one turns to children, the power differential between the data controller imposing standard terms of consent – for example, a school, or a social work agency, or a general practitioner clinic – and the child as data subject becomes even greater. A further problem with consent is, for *how long* does it last? ICO guidance makes it clear that consent once given may not last forever. Combined with the rules restricting data retention, in most cases it seems reasonable to assume that both consent and data should last only as long as necessary for the processing (ICO, undated (a), para 3.1.5, pp 29-30).

Guidance about how consent should be *obtained* can also be drawn from the other requirements in the 1998 DPA for 'fair processing'. First, when considering if processing is 'fair', regard must be had to the method by which consent is obtained. For example, it will not be 'fair' if the data subject was deceived or misled (1998 DPA, Schedule 1, Part II, para 1(1)). Second, the data subject giving consent must be given information as far as is practicable at the appropriate time about the identity of the data controller, and the *purposes* for which the data are being collected. In general, those purposes should be made public and specific in the register where data controllers are required to make an entry and which is available via the Information Commissioner's website. However, as has been noted by commentators, these purposes are often specified in very broad terms and even the standard categories for notification provided by the Information Commissioner do little to prevent such broad categories being selected. For example, it is legitimate to say little more than that data are being collected or processed for reasons such as 'research' or 'education' (Anderson et al, 2006). Among private sector data collectors, it is common to register so many categories of reasons for data collection, that few if any categories of data collected will be potentially left out and so 'unfairly' processed.

When do children acquire *capacity* to consent under the 1998 DPA? In Scotland, this is specified in the 1998 DPA (section 66): consent can be given by a child under 16 as soon as he (or she) has a 'general understanding' of what it means to exercise the right to give consent. A person aged 12 or over is presumed to be of sufficient age and maturity to have that capacity. Below that age, the person or persons with parental responsibilities and rights should in principle give consent.[10]

In England, the situation is less clear. The ICO has not provided specific guidance and the Act is silent. In principle, drawing on the seminal child capacity case of *Gillick v West Norfolk and Wisbech AHA*,[11] it would appear that a child should have the ability to give consent to data collection or processing when he (or she) is of an age and maturity to understand the nature and consequences of exercising that capacity. This is the standard test for the giving of medical consent by a child without the consent (and in some cases, the knowledge) of his parent or guardian and has become known as 'Gillick competence'. However, as the writers of the FIPR report on children's databases (Anderson et al, 2006) have observed, the interpretation of *Gillick* is also not entirely straightforward, a point returned to later. Again, if a child is not 'Gillick competent', it seems that data protection rights should be exercised for the child by those with parental responsibilities and rights.

Exemptions

A number of important exemptions from and modifications to the 1998 DPA exist, either as provisions in the Act itself or in separate statutory instruments. The exemptions in the 1998 DPA can be found in Part IV (sections 28-36) and Schedule 7. These exemptions either apply to the subject information provisions[12] or the non-disclosure provisions.[13] They are wide ranging and include, for example:

- National security (1998 DPA, section 28);
- Crime and taxation (1998 DPA, section 29);
- Research, history and statistics (1998 DPA, section 33);
- Disclosures required by law and in connection with legal proceedings (1998 DPA, section 35(1));
- Exemptions contained within the Data Protection (Miscellaneous Subject Access Exemptions) Order 2000;[14]
- Orders made in relation to health, education and social work (1998 DPA, section 30):
  - Health (the Data Protection [Subject Access Modification] [Health] Order 2000);[15]
  - Education (the Data Protection [Subject Access Modifications] [Education] Order 2000);[16]
  - Social Work (the Data Protection [Subject Access Modifications] [Social Work] Order 2000);[17]

- Legal professional privilege
- Self-incrimination.

Data protection and the 2000 Freedom of Information Act and 2002 Freedom of Information (Scotland) Act

The Freedom of Information (FOI) Acts seek to encourage openness and greater public accountability by facilitating access to information held by public authorities. Both Acts provide that any person, legal or natural, has a right to know whether information, either about himself or a third party, of a particular kind is held by a public authority and to have that information communicated. The public authority concerned has to reasonably accommodate the applicant. The request for information has to be in writing and the applicant has to sufficiently identify himself and pay the prescribed fees. The FOI Act interacts with the 1998 DPA in that a request made under FOI can be refused if it relates to 'personal data'. The data subject alone has subject access rights to those data, and has not consented to anyone else seeing those data. It would interfere with his or her informational privacy if anyone could obtain access via an FOI request.

This interaction is already reportedly causing considerable difficulty, as already seen in the Scottish FOI case of *Common Services Agency v Scottish Information Commissioner*.[18] In that case, difficulties arose because information that related to patients treated for childhood leukaemia in Dumfries and Galloway was sought under FOI provisions. Although the information had been anonymised, it was claimed that due to the small numbers involved the information could be traced as 'personal data'. On appeal, however, this argument was dismissed in favour of a liberal interpretation of FOI law.

Confidentiality and breach of confidence law

An obligation of confidence historically arose in principle in two circumstances: one, in a commercial situation where 'trade secrets' were disclosed, and second, where an obligation of confidence was implied by the existence of a recognised relationship of 'trust', for example between solicitor and client, or doctor and patient. If confidence was breached, an action for damages would be possible. Breach of confidence in such circumstances would also usually be a serious breach of professional ethics, which might lead, for example, to a doctor being struck off the medical register.

Since the leading case of *Douglas v Hello!*,[19] however, the law of confidence has been significantly widened by the courts. In that case, it was held that if someone has information that is 'private or personal', and to which he could properly deny access to third parties, and he reasonably intended to profit commercially by using or publishing that information, *then* a third party who is, or ought to be, aware of these matters, and who has knowingly obtained the information without authority, will be in breach of duty if he uses or publishes that information to the detriment of the owner.

Douglas v Hello! was strongly influenced by Article 8 of the ECHR and in subsequent cases the English courts have gone further and used the developing breach of confidence jurisprudence to introduce something almost like a general right of privacy for 'celebrities'. The exact nature and even existence of this right is much contested.[20] Since few children are celebrities, however, this aspect of the law of confidence, although intriguing, is perhaps not yet of much relevance to them. If this string of cases gives rise eventually to a general law of privacy, either in common law or in legislation, however, this may be highly significant to the rights of ordinary folk. An act of disclosure of private information may be a breach of both data protection and the law of confidence; this was true in the case of *Campbell v MGN*[21] where photos published of Naomi Campbell the supermodel, indicating that she was attending Narcotics Anonymous, gave rise to claims for infringement of both regimes.

More germane to children involved with social services is the more traditional notion of confidentiality as something owed by a professional to his (or her) client. This duty will apply to a social worker, a doctor and a teacher. Two issues make this a problematic right for children: first, as above, when do they acquire capacity to exercise a right to confidentiality? Second, what is the impact on this right if others, such as parents or social workers or the police, claim they need to invade the child's privacy to protect his welfare or protect him from risk of abuse?

In relation to capacity, the same issues recur as discussed above in relation to data protection law and consent. Mason and McCall-Smith (1999) confirm that the question of when to respect a child's right to confidentiality again depends on whether that child can be regarded as Gillick competent.[22] However, even if this test is met, there are exceptional circumstances in which a professional such as a doctor may still have the right and/or duty to disclose a child's confidences. The most important of these circumstances is, of course, where a child reveals evidence of abuse. In such a case, public interest demands disclosure and this has been upheld repeatedly in the courts.[23] Although this seems like the obvious balance to strike, it will not be at all easy to carry out in practice without either losing the trust of the child or running a risk of leaving that child in a vulnerable position.[24]

Brayne and Carr (2002b, p 241) comment: 'Public interest, the general justification for disclosure, is a slippery concept, particularly for social workers whose role ranges from caring to the investigation of harmful, often criminal activities'. As they also emphasise, a professional's assessment of whether to conceal or reveal must now be explicitly made having consideration to the 1998 Human Rights Act, and the child's right to respect for private and family life in Article 8. This right, however, is not absolute, and Article 8(1) allows that confidentiality and privacy may be breached to protect 'public safety, for the prevention of disorder or crime, for the protection of health and morals, or for the protection of the rights and freedoms of others'. Public interest confers immunity from redress on the person who discloses: in *D v NSPCC*,[25] an informer who disclosed information of a child protection nature about a child to social workers was entitled not to be identified as part of public interest immunity, even though she had in fact disclosed out of malice rather than a sense of duty.

The 'database nation' for children?

The UK is experiencing a boom in public sector databases devoted – either exclusively or partly – to collecting children's details, including: the National Pupil Database; lost pupil databases; law enforcement databases (where both victims' and offenders' details are recorded); and databases for families and children involved with social services concerning issues such as temporary housing. These have given rise to a number of concerns (ICO, 2006b). As the ICO (2006b, p 5) put it, 'It is hard to imagine any households with children remaining untouched by at least one of the various databases that are being compiled'. Concerns about this evolving children's 'database nation' include possible entrenched discrimination of 'labelled' children, replacement of effective social intervention by 'e-surveillance', sloppy or over-loose interpretation of data protection and privacy law by agencies involved in building these databases, and possibly consequent harm to children either by over- or under-concern (Anderson et al, 2006). The perceived risk here comes not just from the existence of each database, but from the possibility of combining data derived from combinations of these databases, and the risk of turning unsubstantiated inferences or opinions in one database into recorded facts assumed to be true in another.

ContactPoint

Much of the current discontent about whether children are the subject of too much electronic information gathering has found a focus in a FIPR report (Anderson et al, 2006) on what was formerly known as the 'Children's ID Database' and at the time of writing is known as 'ContactPoint'. As McGhee outlines in Chapter Eight in this volume, in England, section 12 of the 2004 Children Act has ushered in a legal framework for the creation of a large integrated database system known technically as the Information Sharing Index, and aimed, according to its accompanying literature, at safeguarding the welfare of children as well as reducing risk of abuse. The Index, when implemented,[26] is intended to contain basic details of all children in England, together with contact details of all practitioners who have provided or are currently providing social and other services to those children (except 'sensitive' services such as mental health services, which are subject to a tighter regime of disclosure). Practitioners may also be able to have it recorded on the Index that they have important information to share, although the details of this provision are to be fleshed out in statutory instruments and remain unclear at the time of writing.

The ostensible aim presented in the consultation period is that the database is intended to promote sharing of information and interagency cooperation, and to enhance child protection and reduce risk of harm to children. In particular it was intended to prevent the kind of well-publicised tragedies such as the death of Victoria Climbié – occasions where information was not shared between agencies until after a child had died or suffered severe harm. These seem indubitably positive and desirable aims.

A more cynical view, however, might be that in the wake of public opposition to a mandatory, single, joined-up, national ID database for adults,[27] the government has turned instead to creating such a database by stealth, by placing all the children of England onto a database. This point has particular relevance when combined with the growing pressure towards putting the entire population on a DNA database from birth. Once information has been gathered on the population since childhood, it may well be difficult to 'un-gather' that information. A less conspiratorial but still negative view might be taken that the extensive resources involved in creating the ContactPoint database might well be better spent on services directly improving or safeguarding the welfare of children. There is also concern that the Index may be used wrongly to label children as potential future criminals or delinquents.[28]

From a *legal* perspective, the key controversial issue is consent to information sharing by the child. The information held on databases like ContactPoint is personal data about the child, and thus by data protection law the child as data subject should have the right to give or withhold consent to that information being processed, stored and shared. The FIPR report view (Anderson et al, 2006) is that children are too routinely asked to consent to giving personal data away without enough guidance, information or protection. In particular, the report asserts that *Gillick*[29] only authorises a child to give consent to information sharing if every effort has been made to involve the parents and that 'where there is no conflict of interest, there is no reason or necessity and therefore no justification, for dispensing with parental consent or involvement' (p 92).

In the context of opposition to a database, which might have harmful effects on both the nation's privacy and children's social services, this attitude is understandable. But it is not wholly compatible with the House of Lords reasoning behind the *Gillick* decision in 1985, and the subsequent development of child law over the last 20 years. *Gillick* was a landmark case, which recognised for the first time the autonomy of the mature minor; it was a sea-change from the preceding law where a child was entirely subject to parental power until he attained majority at 18. *Gillick* has since remained a beacon, despite repeated pressure from litigants and pressure groups, for the rights of autonomous mature minors to obtain, for example, contraceptive services, without direct parental involvement.

In terms of hard law, the FIPR report (Anderson et al, 2006) justifies its interpretation of *Gillick* by concentrating on the speech of Lord Fraser who, famously, incorporated both the welfare principle and the wishes of parents into his ratio for deciding when a mature minor was competent to give consent. Yet less stress is placed on the equally well-known speech of Lord Scarman, who opined that a child had capacity to consent if he (or she) were of sufficient maturity to understand the nature and consequences of what he was consenting to, and made no requirement that the parents be consulted (although it remained extremely desirable), or that the child should act in his best interests. Where there was a conflict of interest between the rights of the parents and that of the child, the child's rights would prevail. In Scotland, Lord Scarman's simpler formulation has formed the basis of the statutory law on medical consent for children in section 2(4) of the 1991 Age of Legal Capacity (Scotland) Act, and has also informed the NHS guidelines on consent for children (Edwards and Griffiths, 2006, p 52). It seems logical in Scotland at least that Lord Scarman's approach be followed in relation to consent to information sharing, rather than Lord Fraser's.

In terms of policy, the question is whether it would be a good thing for children to be asked to consult with their parents in all or almost all cases before agreeing to disclose or share personal information. This may be so, given the complex future risks of information sharing. However, there is a risk of prejudice to their rights of confidentiality and to be treated as emerging young adults in important venues like school, or a doctor's surgery. Children might choose instead not to share information they did not want their parents to know about that could potentially serve as a warning of risk to social services. They might choose not to see professionals in case their parents found out. Anecdotal experience shows that children strongly resent having their confidentiality disrespected and will not reveal information if they fear it will be disclosed without their consent. In part because of this, the Scottish courts have been reluctant to breach the confidentiality of even quite young children giving evidence in family proceedings in court.[30] There are issues also of children's own rights to privacy under Article 8 of the ECHR: children have rights to keep secrets from parents as well as from the state.

Rather than requiring that parents be asked to give consent to information sharing in all cases, a better approach might be to have an independent adult available to advise a child before he or she gave consent to information sharing; a guidance teacher in school perhaps, or the equivalent of a patient's advocate in a hospital or social work environment. Schools might also give a general briefing to their pupils about the nature and risks of information sharing. Such an approach would respect the status of the *Gillick*-competent minor while protecting them from risk.

Finally, two further points might be made about this whole debate. One is that discussing who has the right to give consent is something of an academic red herring. Most people, adults or otherwise, give consents to using their personal data to public sector officials all the time without giving a moment's thought to the consequences. The Information Commissioner was recently asked to intervene to stop schools routinely taking fingerprints of children and using them for purposes such as controlling access to library books (*The Register*, 2007a). Would parents have been any more likely than children to have opposed the forces of authority, and refused consent to what appeared a harmless way to stop valuable books being stolen?

Second, the debate around consent focuses too much on *initial* consent to collection of data and not sufficiently on what happens to that information *subsequently*: who gets access to it, who gets to disseminate it, who makes sure the data stay up to date and secure, who decides how long the data are kept? The FIPR report (Anderson et al, 2006) draws attention, correctly, to the fact that much public sector data sharing is legitimised without clear consent by special 'statutory gateways': statutory provisions in administrative law, which, the report argues, are over-broad and do not confer the specific powers used by local authorities and others to share and process data (p 96; citing, for example, the 2000 Local Government Act, section 2). This may be true, but will the response to any challenge not be to pass further more specific laws? The answers here again probably lie not in the minutiae of consent and data protection law but in better procedures to ensure that the policies *behind* data protection law are clearer to data subjects; there is better guidance and procedures for the professionals involved; better education for all concerned; and an increased use of privacy impact assessments when databases are initially proposed and implemented.[31] Such assessments need not be costly and could be undertaken at a very minimal and sensible level; for example, as the ICO said in the library fingerprint debacle cited earlier, schools could have simply used pupils' names, perhaps backed by their student cards, rather than collecting fingerprints, a piece of data whose storage might later be abused.

Final thoughts

This chapter provides a brief outline of data protection law and the law of confidentiality in the UK. What also needs to be fully conveyed is the formalistic nature of talking about privacy rights for children in isolation from the rights of parents, the welfare principle, and the institutional power of the professionals they become involved with in a social services context. The debate in the FIPR Report (Anderson et al, 2006) about whether children should be able to give away information via their own capacity to consent, or whether their parents should be involved, mirrors the debate in children's rights generally about the clash between paternalism and protection (Marshall 1997). The debate about breaching children's confidentiality in the public interest emphasises that children's rights in practice are always contingent on what others (parents, doctors, social workers, courts, governments) see as in their best interests.

Children in general have neither the knowledge nor the power to enforce their own rights. As is true of data subjects and data protection law generally, children will only have their privacy protected if a culture of compliance emerges by self-regulation of the players with power – the public sector data controllers. The FIPR report is valuable in highlighting the issue of the dangers of widespread sharing of child-related information without adequate safeguards and foresight as to future risks. However, the solution lies less with the minutiae of consent and amending local government information sharing powers, than with the creation of a privacy-compliant culture for the public sector, effectively watch-dogged by a properly resourced ICO. In this context, the introduction by the Information Commissioner of a Code on Information Sharing (ICO, 2007) is a significant response, even though it does not change any substantive law. The outcomes of a major consultation launched by the government on public data sharing are expected during 2008 (Thomas and Walport, 2007).

Second, rights to privacy appear to be more readily ignored when transferred into the digital, information society world than when exercised in the familiar offline environment. Most people would be fairly annoyed if someone followed them around all day with a camcorder. Yet until recently, the population of the UK expressed either little interest or actual positive approval at the appearance of a CCTV camera on almost every street in the UK.[32] Similar effects can be seen when we talk about children and technology. In Tokyo, school children are routinely tagged with radio-frequency identification (RFID) tags, so that parents can monitor them wherever they go. This is often reported with apparent approval and no conception of what it means to the children to be locatable '24/7' (Swedberg, 2005).

Finally, it is worth noting that although the focus of this book is information sharing in the public sector (primarily social and health services), the threat to children's privacy may in future come more from the *private* sector than from the state (see Steeves, 2006). Data of an extremely sensitive nature are extensively collected from and about children of increasingly young ages as they interact on online social networking sites like Bebo, Club Penguin, MySpace and FaceBook, to name but a few. Children and young people freely give away their most intimate secrets on sites like these: social, sexual and emotional secrets are shared with amazing (or appalling) ease. The privacy settings on such sites are often either non-existent or not easy to use, which means that such information may be effectively broadcast to the world, and then indexed in search engines.[33] The full implications of this culture of disclosure rather than secrecy may yet be seen when these children come of age where they are looking for jobs and life partners, and discover that their embarrassing past has been published and indexed in glorious detail on Google.

Notes

[1] EC: 108th Convention for the protection of individuals concerning automatic processing of personal data (1981).

[2] Directive 95/46/EC of the European Parliament and of the Council of 24 October 1995 on the protection of individuals with regard to the processing of personal data and on the free movement of such data.

[3] G.A. res. 217A (III), U.N. Doc A/810 at 71 (1948).

[4] G.A. res. 2200A (XXI), 21 U.N. GAOR Supp. (No. 16) at 52, U.N. Doc. A/6316 (1966), 999 U.N.T.S. 171, entered into force 23 March 1976.

[5] *Official Journal L 281, 23/11/1995 P. 0031-0050.*

[6] For exemptions and restrictions, see DPD, Article 13.

[7] See interpretation of 'relevant filing system' in *Durant v FSA* [2003] EWCA Civ 1746, Court of Appeal (Civil Division).

[8] Note 7 above. The meaning of personal data in the context of anonymised medical data was also discussed in the Scottish FOI case, *Common Services Agency v Scottish Information Commissioner* [2006] CSIH 58, www.scotcourts.gov.uk/opinions/2006CSIH58.html (this case is currently under appeal to the House of Lords).

[9] See, however, *Johnson v Medical Defence Union Ltd* [2007] EWCA Civ 26 for a case where an activity was not held to be 'processing' within the DPA scheme.

[10] This arises from the general law relating to parental responsibilities and rights: see the 1995 Children (Scotland) Act, sections 1 and 2. This rule is modified by specific rules in statutory instruments, eg the Data Protection (Subject Access Modification) (Social Work) Order 2000, SI 2000/415, provides that a parent cannot make a subject access request on behalf of a child if it would be likely to prejudice the carrying on of social work by virtue of resultant serious harm to the child or another person. Similar rules exist in relation to health data (SI 2000/413) and education data (SI 2000/414).

[11] [1985] 3 All ER 402.

[12] Paragraphs 2 and 3 of Part II of Schedule I of the Act (fair processing of information) and section 7, subject access.

[13] The First Data Protection Principle, except where it requires compliance with the conditions in Schedules 2 and 3 of the Act (the conditions for processing and conditions for processing sensitive data); the Second, Third, Fourth and Fifth Data Protection Principles; section 10 (right to prevent processing likely to cause damage or distress); and sections 14(1) to (3) (rectification, blocking, erasure and destruction).

[14] SI 2000/419 (as amended by the Data Protection (Miscellaneous Subject Access Exemptions) (Amendment) Order, SI 2000/1865.

[15] SI 2000/413, also called the 'Health Order'.

[16] SI 2000/414, the 'Education Order'.

[17] SI 2000/415, the 'Social Work Order'.

[18] Above note 8.

[19] [2005] EWCA Civ 595.

[20] See, in particular, *Campbell v MGN* [2002] EWCA Civ 1373; *McGregor v Fraser* [2003] EWHC 2972; *Ash v McKennit* [2005] EWHC 3003 (QB).

[21] Above note 20.

[22] See also Brayne and Carr (2002a), Part 1, at p 166, n 2.

[23] See, for example, *L v UK* [2000] 2 FCR 145 (European Court of Human Rights upheld the right of police to access evidence of abuse of children by heroin-addicted parents, even though the information was subject to expert witness privilege). General Medical Council guidelines also specifically allow a doctor to break confidentiality in cases of abuse (*Confidentiality: Protecting and Providing Information,* April 2004, para 29, www.gmc-uk.org/guidance/current/library/confidentiality.asp, cf *W v Egdell* [1990] Ch 359).

[24] See further the controversial case of *W v Egdell* [1990] Ch 359 (a case involving duty of confidence owed by a psychiatrist to an adult patient).

[25] [1978] AC 171.

[26] The 2007 Children Act 2004 Information Database (England) Regulations, SI 2007/2182 were passed on 24 July 2007 to implement section 12 of the 2007 Act. Commentary can be found on the website of the independent watchdog body ARCH (www.arch-ed.org/). The House of Lords Committee on the Merits of Statutory Instruments criticised the ContactPoint database severely in their debate on 17 July 2007, implying that it might be disproportionate in terms of the ECHR human right to privacy. Following the HMRC Child Benefit data leak, the launch of ContactPoint has been delayed to October 2008 to allow for a review of security processes.

[27] See BBC News, 'Giant ID computer plan scrapped', 19 December 2006, http://news.bbc.co.uk/1/hi/uk_politics/6192419.stm

[28] Further arguments on ContactPoint can be found both at the ARCH website, www.arch-ed.org/issues/databases/IS%20Index.htm, and in the FIPR report (Anderson et al, 1996). The ICO itself expresses worries about the Index in its Issues Paper (ICO, 2006b).

[29] Above note 11.

[30] See *McGrath v McGrath* 1999 SLT (Sh Ct) 86; *Dosoo v Dosoo* 1999 SLT (Sh Ct) 86.

[31] See Ashe, Chapter Nine, this volume.

[32] See further Goold (2004), discussed in Edwards (2005).

[33] See discussion on the author's blog of FaceBook and its lack of privacy and security, http://blogscript.blogspot.com/2007/06/facebook-brought-to-book.html

References

Anderson, R., Brown, I., Clayton, R., Dowty, T., Korff, D. and Munro, E. (2006) *Children's Databases – Safety and Privacy: A Report for the Information Commissioner*, Foundation for Information Policy Research, www.ico.gov.uk/upload/documents/library/data_protection/detailed_specialist_guides/ico_issues_paper_protecting_chidrens_personal_information.pdf (the 'FIPR report').

BBC News (2007) 'Child database system postponed', 27 November, http://news.bbc.co.uk/1/hi/education/7115546.stm

Bennett, C. J. and Raab, C. (2006) *The Governance of Privacy: Policy Instruments in Global Perspective* (2nd edn), Cambridge, MA: MIT Press.

Brayne, H. and Carr, H. (2002a) 'Confidentiality, secrecy, children and human rights, part 1: keeping the lid on', *Representing Children*, vol 15, no 3, pp 152-68.

Brayne, H. and Carr, H. (2002b) 'Confidentiality, secrecy, children and human rights, part 2: lifting the lid', *Representing Children*, vol 15, no 4, pp 241-57.

Busch, A. (2006) 'From safe harbour to the rough sea? Privacy disputes across the Atlantic', *SCRIPT-ed*, vol 3, no 4, 304, www.law.ed.ac.uk/ahrc/script-ed/vol3-4/busch.asp

Bygrave, L. (2002) *Data Protection Law: Approaching its Rationale, Logic and Limits*, Information Law Series-10, The Hague: Kluwer Law International

Carey, P. (2004) *Data Protection: A Practical Guide to UK and EU Law* (2nd edition), Oxford: Oxford University Press.

Edwards, L. (2005) 'Switching off the surveillance society? Legal regulation of CCTV in the UK', in S. Nouwt, B. R. deVries and C. Prins (eds) *Reasonable Expectations of Privacy? Eleven Country Reports on Camera Surveillance and Workplace Privacy*, The Hague: TMC Asser Press, pp 91-114.

Edwards, L. and Griffiths, A. (2006) *Family Law* (2nd edition), Edinburgh: Thomson/W. Green.

EU Article 29 Data Protection Working Party (2008) *Working Document 1/2008 on the Protection of Children's Personal Data*, WP147, http://ec.europa.eu/justice_home/fsj/privacy/docs/wpdocs/2008/wp147_en.pdf

Garfinkel, S. (2001) *Database Nation: The Death of Privacy in the 21st Century*, Cambridge, MA: O'Reilly.

Goold, B. J. (2004) *CCTV and Policing: Public Area Surveillance and Police Practices in Britain*, Clarendon studies in criminology, Oxford: Oxford University Press.

HM Treasury (2007) 'Terms of reference for the Poynter Review', Press notice, www.hm-treasury.gov.uk./newsroom_and_speeches/press/2007/press_133_07.cfm

ICO (Information Commissioners Office) (2006a) *What Price Privacy Now?*, www.ico.gov.uk/upload/documents/library/corporate/research_and_reports/ico-wppnow-0602.pdf

ICO (2006b) *Protecting Children's Personal Information: ICO Issues Paper*, 22 November, www.ico.gov.uk/upload/documents/library/data_protection/detailed_specialist_guides/issues_paper_protecting_childrens_personal_information.pdf

Information Commissioners Office (2007) *Framework Code of Practice for Sharing Personal Information*, August, www.ico.gov.uk/upload/documents/library/data_protection/detailed_specialist_guides/pinfo-framework.pdf

ICO (undated (a)) *Data Protection Act 1998: Legal Guidance*, www.ico.gov.uk/upload/documents/library/data_protection/detailed_specialist_guides/data_protection_act_legal_guidance.pdf

ICO (undated (b)) Data Protection document library, www.ico.gov.uk/tools_and_resources/document_library/data_protection.aspx

JCHR (Joint Committee on Human Rights) (2008) *Data Protection and Human Rights: Fourteenth Report of Session 2007-08*, HC 132, London: The Stationery Office, www.publications.parliament.uk/pa/jt200708/jtselect/jtrights/72/72.pdf

Marshall, K. (1997) *Children's Rights in the Balance: The Participation-Protection Debate*, Edinburgh: The Stationery Office.

Mason, J.K. and McCall-Smith, R.A. (1999) *Law and Medical Ethics* (5th edition), London: Butterworths.

Rosen, J. (2001) *The Unwanted Gaze: The Destruction of Privacy in America*, New York: Vintage Books.

Steeves, V. (2006) 'It's not child's play: the online invasion of children's privacy', *University of Ottawa Law and Technology Journal*, vol 169, www.uoltj.ca

Swedberg, C. (2005) 'RFID Watches Over School Kids in Japan: a group of children in Yokohama City wears active tags to keep them safe on their way to and from school', *RFID Journal*, www.rfidjournal.com/article/articleview/2050/1/1/

The Register (2007a) 'Info Commissioner: too late to stop school fingerprinting', 17 January, www.theregister.co.uk/2007/01/17/fingerprinting_bolted/

Thomas, R. and Walport, M. (2007) 'Data sharing review. A consultation paper on the use and sharing of personal information in the public and private sector', www.justice.gov.uk/reviews/datasharing-intro.htm

Wood, D.M. (ed) (2006) *A Report on the Surveillance Society for the Information Commissioner*, Surveillance Studies Network, www.ico.gov.uk/upload/documents/library/data_protection/practical_application/surveillance_society_full_report_2006.pdf

Public protection in practice: Multi-Agency Public Protection Arrangements (MAPPA)

Hazel Kemshall and Jason Wood[1]

Introduction

The late 1990s saw the development of Multi-Agency Public Protection Arrangements (MAPPA) in England and Wales (with slightly later developments in Scotland). These arrangements were given legislative force in the 2000 Criminal Justice and Courts Services Act (sections 67 and 68), with police, probation (and prisons added by the 2003 Criminal Justice Act; CJA) as 'responsible authorities' tasked with risk assessing and managing offenders who meet the MAPPA criteria (Home Office, 2004). In order to carry out these duties, personal information on offenders is collected, stored and exchanged. MAPPA agencies are mindful that they must operate within the law, particularly the European Convention on Human Rights (ECHR) and data protection legislation; but also that key inquiries (for example Bichard, 2004) and high-profile cases have highlighted the difficulties for appropriate risk assessment and management occasioned by failures to exchange information between relevant agencies. This chapter will explore the types of personal information required for effective risk assessment and risk management; and how it is reviewed, used and exchanged. The tensions around individual and third party confidentiality (for example victim information) will be reviewed, and also disclosure to agencies within MAPPA and to affected third parties (for example schools).

Accountability processes for appropriate information management, including the transparency of decision making and third party disclosure, will be addressed, and also issues of monitoring and surveillance (often covert) of high-risk offenders. The discussion will draw on three evaluation studies involving the authors (Maguire et al, 2001; Kemshall et al, 2005; Wood and Kemshall, 2007), utilising direct observation of panel meetings, discussion with MAPPA representatives, interviews with offenders, and case file reading. In addition, key literature and recent inquiries will be drawn on, most notably the Bichard inquiry following the Soham murders, the Hanson and White Serious Further Offence report (HMIP, 2006a), and the report into the murder committed by Anthony Rice (HMIP, 2006b). The chapter will conclude by considering the overall regulation and accountability of the MAPPA system including consistency of practice, standards and the avoidance of abuse.

What *are* MAPPA?

Multi-Agency Public Protection Arrangements (MAPPA) were formally created by sections 67 and 68 of the 2000 Criminal Justice and Courts Services Act, although they had evolved from multiagency arrangements in the late 1990s for the assessment and management of sex offenders subject to the sex offender register. These arrangements were consolidated by the 2003 Criminal Justice Act (CJA) and made police, probation and prisons 'responsible authorities' while giving other agencies a 'duty to cooperate'. These arrangements place a statutory responsibility on the three main agencies to assess and manage high-risk offenders. MAPPA are concerned with three categories of offender:

- Category 1 – Registered sex offenders who have been convicted or cautioned since September 1997 of certain sexual offences (2003 CJA, section 327(2)), and are required to register personal and other relevant details with the police in order to be effectively monitored. The police have primary responsibility for identifying category 1 offenders.
- Category 2 – Violent and other sexual offenders receiving a custodial sentence of 12 months or more, and since April 2001, a hospital or guardianship order, or subject to disqualification from working with children (2003 CJA, section 327(3)-(5)). All these offenders are subject to statutory supervision by the National Probation Service and consequently probation is responsible for the identification of category 2 offenders.
- Category 3 – Other offenders considered by the responsible authority to pose a 'risk of serious harm to the public' (2003 CJA, section 325(2)). Identification is largely determined by the judgement of the responsible authority based on two main considerations:

– The offender must have a conviction that indicates she or he is capable of causing serious harm to the public.

– The responsible authority must reasonably consider that the offender may cause harm to the public. The responsibility of identification lies with the agency that deals initially with the offender. (Home Office, 2004)

MAPPA also have a three-tier pyramid structure, aimed at targeting resources at the highest level of risk or 'critical few':

- Level 1 offenders ('Ordinary risk management') – where the agency responsible for the offender can manage the risk without the significant involvement of other agencies; only appropriate for category 1 and category 2 offenders who are assessed as presenting a low or medium risk.
- Level 2 (Local interagency risk management) – where there is 'active involvement' of more than one agency in risk management plans, either because of a higher level of risk or because of the complexity of managing the offender. Responsible authorities should decide the frequency of panel meetings and also the representation and quality assurance of risk management.
- Level 3 (MAPPP – Multi-Agency Public Protection Panel) – those offenders defined as the 'critical few' who pose a high or very high risk, in addition to having a media profile, and/or management plan drawing together key active partners who will take joint responsibility for the community management of the offender. Level 3 cases can be 'referred down' to Level 2 when risk of harm diminishes. A multi-agency public protection panel is a full meeting of all the agencies working in MAPPA and is used to risk assess the 'critical few' and to agree and review risk management plans. (Home Office, 2004, paras 111-16)

MAPPA have been characterised as a 'community protection model' (Connelly and Williamson, 2000). This model is embedded in the criminal justice system and is characterised by the use of restriction, surveillance, monitoring and control, compulsory treatment and the prioritisation of victim/community rights over those of offenders.

Special measures such as licence conditions, tagging, exclusions, registers and selective incarceration are all extensively used (Kemshall, 2001, 2003; Kemshall et al, 2005). Risk management plans are devised and delivered by statutory agencies in partnership (Home Office, 2004), with police and probation as key drivers (Kemshall, 2003; Nash, 2006), with the Prison Service added as a statutory partner by the 2003 CJA.

Public protection is also a sensitive and contentious issue, attracting much media and political attention since its inception in the early 1990s (Kemshall, 2003). Public protection and risk management failures elicit public scrutiny and blame, resulting in the dismissal of staff and most notably in the resignation of the Home Secretary Charles Clark in 2006. In this climate the focus on appropriate information exchange and disclosure both between agencies and to relevant third parties (including potential victims) has been acute.

MAPPA, information exchange and the meaning of confidentiality

A core task of MAPPA is information exchange between key agencies, notably police, probation and prisons (and often including agencies that have a 'duty to cooperate' such as social services and healthcare) in order to risk assess those offenders referred to them. Such assessments need to be reliable and comprehensive, and as such in-depth information about the offender is required. This information exchange is given statutory force by sections 67 and 68 of the 2000 Criminal Justice and Courts Services Act, and later by the 2003 CJA; and section 115 of the 1998 Crime and Disorder Act, allowing information exchange for the purposes of preventing crime and disorder. The 2003 CJA imposed a 'duty to cooperate' on other key agencies (as previously listed) that may have information pertinent to the risks posed by the offender. As stated in the Home Office Guidance (Home Office, 2004, para 85), this ensures that 'all MAPPA agencies ... have the prima facie legal power to exchange information with the Responsible Authority'.

Paragraph 83 of the Home Office Guidance (2004) states that:

> Information sharing must:
> i)   have lawful authority;
> ii) be necessary;
> iii) be proportionate; and done in ways which,

iv) ensure the safety and security of the information shared; and,

v) be accountable.

MAPPA therefore operate within a climate where information exchange is both legitimated and expected, and the limits to that exchange are in effect set by the principles above. MAPPA are expected to have, and carefully operate, information sharing protocols, which reflect both law and guidance (Kemshall et al, 2005). Exchange is justified on the 'necessary principle', based on the requirement to 'properly assess and manage the risks posed by those offenders who are subject to MAPPA provisions' (Home Office, 2004, para 86), and these requirements are further specified as:

- to identify those offenders who present a serious risk of harm to the public;
- to ensure that the assessment of the risks they present are accurate; and,
- to enable the most appropriate plans to be drawn up and implemented to manage the assessed risks and thereby protect the public. (Home Office, 2004, para 86)

Such information sharing must also be proportionate, driven by the level of the risk of serious harm posed and the needs of other agencies to know about the risk in order to contribute to effective risk management. For example, prisons will now routinely share information within MAPPA, and in particular with police and probation in order to make effective plans for the management of high-risk offenders on release. This is particularly important for those offenders released without parole supervision at the end of their sentence but who are still considered to present a significant risk of harm to the public. In such cases MAPPA may arrange for voluntary contact with probation, police surveillance (often covert), or in the case of high-risk sex offenders applications have been made for Sexual Offences Prevention Orders (SOPOs) (Wood and Kemshall, 2007). (SOPOs can be made in magistrates' courts on the application of the police to prevent further sexual offending by a known sexual offender. They are subject to civil rather than criminal standards of proof, and require the police to provide evidence that a pattern of sexual offending exists and that there is a reasonable risk of further offending.) Exchange of information and subsequent actions are justified on the grounds of public protection and that such offenders meet the MAPPA criteria. Third party disclosure to members of the public or potential victims may also be made in certain circumstances in order to achieve their protection (see page 117 and following for discussion).

Secure data storage is also essential, particularly as much information is exchanged electronically and also stored on agency databases such as the Police National Computer (PNC) or the probation database. A further development is the national implementation in January 2007 of ViSOR – the Violent and Sex Offender Register (Probation Circular 40/2006) – to facilitate storage of data about these offenders, which is accessible (with certain restrictions) to police and probation staff. Probation Circular 40/2006 outlines the rigorous access and data-inputting procedures for ViSOR aimed at ensuring quality and confidentiality. Many MAPPA areas have created local MAPPA databases with restricted access procedures adding to the efficiency of local MAPPA in reviewing cases but also adding to the proliferation of databases on high-risk offenders (Kemshall et al, 2005). This can present some difficulties of duplication, but more importantly the potential for error and conflicting information across agencies. Best practice procedures are developing both to track and audit trail information exchange and also to ensure that only reliable information is stored (Kemshall et al, 2005). Such audit trails also provide evidence that information has only been exchanged and used in an accountable manner and according to both legal and guidance principles.

Kemshall et al (2005) found that the majority of MAPPA areas reported that their information sharing procedures were effective, although the main problem reported was in obtaining information from health-related services, and specifically the potential conflict between patient confidentiality and the need for public safety (a situation still somewhat problematic in the more recent evaluation by Wood and Kemshall [2007]). This reflects to some extent the differing cultural and ideological frames within which personnel in health and criminal justice operate, and also the differing legal and operational requirements that are perceived to apply within these agencies. The Royal College of Psychiatrists suggests that a 'duty to co-operate' does not always imply a duty to share information (Royal College of Psychiatrists, 2004).

Information routinely provided to panels includes Police National Computer (PNC) checks, previous convictions, sex offender (and more recently ViSOR) registration, checks with social services child protection registers, information from victim support and, where appropriate, prison discipline record. This information is often supported by police observations and surveillance, probation records and information from supervising officers, and in some cases information on allegations that did not result in court action. One of the key issues in this kind of information is to establish the reliability and accuracy of information passed (including anecdotal or observational information as opposed to demonstrably factual information). In some areas the police grade information according to reliability of source, accuracy and the extent to which the information has been independently verified or corroborated.

Confidentiality and public protection: the principles of third party disclosure

In discussion with MAPPA personnel it is clear that the overriding principle for information exchange is public protection, and that concerns about confidentiality are set within this clear parameter (Wood and Kemshall, 2007). This is, however, routinely tested by the necessity for third party disclosure and the increased sensitivities particularly if disclosure is to individual members of the public, where there can be less control over how that information is subsequently used or whether its confidentiality will be respected. Such disclosures usually require a detailed consideration of risks to the offender (for example the risk of vigilante action), and a balancing of relative costs and benefits of taking such action. Such third party disclosure is covered in some detail in the Home Office Guidance (Home Office, 2004, paras 93-5), and the essential criteria for such a decision to be made are presented in paragraph 95 (emphasis in original):

    i)   the offender presents *a risk of serious harm* to the person, or to those for whom the recipient of the information has responsibility (children, for example);

    ii)   *there is no other practicable, less intrusive means of protecting the individual(s), and failure to disclose would put them in danger.* Also, only that information which is necessary to prevent the harm may be disclosed, which will rarely be all the information available;

    iii) *the risk to the offender should be considered although it should not outweigh the potential risk to others were disclosure not to be made.* The offender retains his rights (most importantly his Article 2 right to life) and consideration must be given to whether those rights are endangered as a consequence of the disclosure. It is partly in respect of such consideration that widespread disclosure of the identity and whereabouts of an offender is very, very rarely if ever justified;

iv) the *disclosure is to the right person* and that they understand the confidential and sensitive nature of the information they have received. The right person will be the person who needs to know in order to avoid or prevent the risks;

v) *consider consulting the offender* about the proposed disclosure. This should be done in all cases unless to do so would not be safe or appropriate. Where consultation can be done, it can help strengthen the risk management plan. If it is possible and appropriate to obtain the offender's consent then a number of potential objections to the disclosure are overcome. Equally, the offender may wish to leave the placement rather than have any disclosure made, and if this is appropriate, this would also avoid the need for any disclosure;

vi) *ensure that whoever has been given the information knows what to do with it.* Again, where this is a specific person, this may be less problematic but in the case of an employer, for example, you may need to provide advice and support; and

vii) before actually disclosing the information, particularly to an employer or someone in a similar position, *first ask them whether they have any information about the offender.* If they have the information then no disclosure is necessary. If they have some but possibly incorrect information your disclosure can helpfully correct it.

As anticipated these criteria have resulted in few disclosures to individual members of the public, and the spectre of vigilantism is very real. The police in particular are concerned about the public disorder issues arising from disclosures and the necessary diversion of policing resources this entails (Wood and Kemshall, 2007). In recent research MAPPA personnel presented clear practice evidence of good conduct on 'controlled disclosure', that is, the limited third party disclosure allowed by the MAPPA guidance reviewed above (Wood and Kemshall, 2007) and followed the process outlined in Figure 6.1.

Interestingly, most disclosures (to employers, accommodation providers, church groups) are done with the consent of the offender, either by the offender in person at the instigation of the supervising officer, or by the supervisor on the offender's behalf. In interview, offenders are quite aware of the need to disclose, and recognise that this will be routinely done on a 'need to know basis'. Of particular

Figure 6.1: Process for controlled disclosure (best practice)

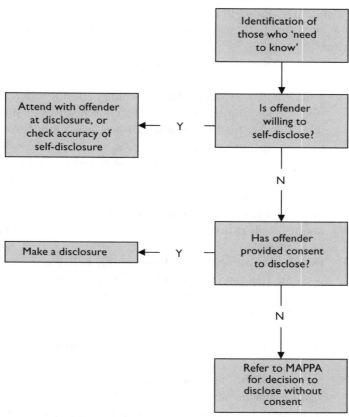

Source: Wood and Kemshall (2007)

note was the effective liaison between some MAPPA and church groups (recognised as a potential site of grooming by sex offenders), resulting in defined procedures for disclosure to church liaison officers to ensure that the church attendance of known paedophiles could be restricted to non-family services. This removed the necessity to tell the whole congregation, but enabled 'chaperoning' by key members of the congregation and restricted access to children. This procedure ensured public safety, informal supervision, some community reintegration and support, and disclosure only on a need to know basis ensuring minimal risk of vigilante action. Such an approach also appears to realistically balance public protection with a limited guarantee of privacy for the offender – a limit that most offenders interviewed understood and accepted.

This controlled disclosure was supported by a contract with the offender reiterating the restrictions on attendance but also the reasons for disclosure – thus, the 'rules' were transparent and accountability clear.

Disclosure is made in a range of circumstances, most notably:

- where there is evidence that grooming behaviours may take place (for example through leisure clubs, churches, employment);
- where others (including other service users) may be at risk (for example in supervised accommodation). It is extremely rare for other service users to be told, but staff and managers are told in order to enable more appropriate placements and for greater vigilance to be exerted;
- to protect past or potential victims (for example, there may be a controlled disclosure to a past victim or relatives indicating release of an offender);
- to schools and colleges if grooming behaviours need to be prevented. In the case of young offenders, limited and controlled disclosure may be made to school or college staff. (Wood and Kemshall, 2007)

Controlled disclosure needs to be handled sensitively, and requires:

- preparation and discussion with those receiving the information;
- an informed decision (via the MAPPA) as to what level of disclosure is required. For example, this might be about the risk factors but not necessarily cover all of the offender's offence history;
- covering the key triggers for offending behaviour and the requirements for successful risk management. 'This is what you need to look out for...'; 'If you see X you need to do Y';
- mechanisms and procedures for support (for example, rapid telephone contact with key personnel/supervising officers via mobile phones). (Wood and Kemshall, 2007)

MAPPA personnel and supervising officers in police and probation were consistent in their view that this approach was effective. In particular, it was seen to reduce anxiety in those who were told, and those receiving the information were clear as to what to do and why, and who else they could or could not disclose to.

The case for wider public disclosure: the usefulness of 'Megan's Law'

The case for public disclosure of high-risk offenders in the community, euphemistically known as 'Megan's Law' (Petrunik, 2003), gained much ground after the murder of Sarah Payne in 2000 resulted in a campaign for a 'Sarah's Law'. Evaluations in the US (Lovell, 2001; Thomas, 2003) have presented a mixed picture of the benefits of disclosure with inconclusive evidence for the impact of disclosure on public safety levels (see also Nash, 2006). In addition, the high levels of sex offender compliance with registration requirements (currently 97% in England and Wales) are in marked contrast to the US figure, which is between 10% and 40% lower (Nash, 2006, p 138). Researchers and professionals attribute these different figures to the differences in public notification (Elbogen et al, 2003; Thomas, 2003; Nash, 2006). In their research, Wood and Kemshall (2007) found that MAPPA personnel saw public disclosure as counterproductive. Indeed, in some cases where offenders had been identified and targeted by members of the public, this had resulted in very difficult and resource-costly public disorder incidents. Offenders also opposed public disclosure, fearing it would result in extreme persecution and make compliance with treatment, monitoring and residence requirements difficult. This resonates with the findings from research in the US (Lovell, 2001).

In November 2006 a limited public disclosure was introduced enabling the release of information, with the approval of the Chief Constable, about 'missing' high-risk offenders, and the 'most wanted' list is published online by the Child Exploitation and Online Protection (CEOP) Centre (see www.crimestoppers-uk.org/ceop/). This development resulted in a limited public and media discussion of the implications for the rights of offenders, although the general tenor of the discussion was that offender rights had a justifiably lower priority than public or victim safety (a view echoed in the US – see Thomas, 2003; Nash, 2006). Indeed, the discussion of human rights (set in the UK within the ECHR legislation) has tended to bemoan the overemphasis on offender rights at the expense of public protection or victim safety, epitomised by the White Paper *Rebalancing the Criminal Justice System in Favour of the Law Abiding Majority: Cutting Crime, Reducing Reoffending and Protecting the Public* (Home Office, 2006a; see also Home Office, 2006b).

Notwithstanding current judicial challenges by offenders under ECHR legislation, politicians (and indeed some senior policy makers) have contended that practitioners have given undue weight to the human rights of offenders at the compromise of public safety. Such criticisms largely began with the Bichard inquiry (2004) following the murders of Holly Wells and Jessica Chapman at Soham in August 2003. The key issue was the employment of their murderer Ian Huntley as a school caretaker even though Huntley had been interviewed (without charge) over the suspected commission of sexual offences. This information was not disclosed to the local education authority or the school, and not transmitted between police services. In brief, in a large document containing some 31 recommendations, Bichard not only instigated a more rigorous system for the vetting of those working with children (see Nash, 2006, p 143 for an interesting discussion on this), but also moved the balance away from individual rights to privacy to public protection, especially where vulnerable victims such as children are concerned. Enhanced disclosures for those working with or having access to children can now include intelligence as well as facts, and allegations as well as convictions. Bichard also recommended greater clarity and training for practitioners on the content of the 1998 Data Protection Act, contending that it had been misapplied in Huntley's case. As Nash (2006, p 144) notes, the Bichard inquiry also raised issues with the quality of police inputting of data, a position that had not improved by the time of Bichard's interim report on progress. This issue arose again in respect of Britons committing sexual offences abroad in January 2007 (see BBC Online, 2007).

Further contentions that human rights concerns had been misapplied were raised in 2006 by Her Majesty's Chief Inspector of Probation in the Serious Further Offence report on Anthony Rice, who committed murder while on release from prison on a life licence (HMIP, 2006b; see also HMIP, 2006a). This case also raised issues about the appropriate balance between offender and (potential) victim. It was contended that EHCR Article 8 (the right to respect for privacy and family life) and Article 11 (the right to freedom of assembly and association) were violated by the residence, exclusion and curfew conditions (see HMIP, 2006b, for a full discussion). However, such rights can be limited by the necessity to protect others, especially if the limits are proportionate to the risk of harm presented (HMIP, 2006b).

The general trend, then, is for protection of the public to outweigh individual rights, although judicial reviews and challenges continue. The key test is proportionality and necessity, and, as importantly, the processes by which such disclosures are made and to whom.

Surveillance versus privacy

A growing feature of risk management has been the use of surveillance, both overt and covert, to gather further information on offenders (about grooming behaviours, victim targeting strategies) and to monitor compliance with risk management plans (for example that exclusion zones or curfews are being observed). Details of surveillance mechanisms are withheld here to preserve the integrity of ongoing and future operations. However, such strategies can include electronic tagging, satellite tracking (to monitor compliance with exclusions and curfews), staff observations and nightly checks in hostels, and unannounced visits and observations by police and probation staff. Again, challenges have been raised under Article 8 (currently under judicial review), and as in the Rice case referred to earlier, such 'restrictive conditions' can be seen by the offender as over-intrusive and unjustified. While legal rulings are awaited, the principles of necessity and proportionality are commonly applied by MAPPA to decide surveillance strategies and it is likely that these are the principles that courts will test. In some instances offenders are told that they will be subject to some form of surveillance and 'checking'. For the most part, offenders recognise the need for this and in some cases feel that such strategies help to 'keep them on track' (Wood and Kemshall, 2007, p 7). The availability of particular technologies, notably satellite and electronic tagging, CCTV, and other forms of electronic monitoring such as key fob logging, have all helped to frame risk management as surveillance and containment. They are relatively cheap, they can be administered by non-professional staff (even contracted out), and compliance with (or breach of) the risk management plan is straightforward (either the offender has violated the exclusion zone or he has not).

In practice, MAPPA make use of two forms of surveillance, characterised here as 'soft surveillance' and 'technologies of surveillance'. Both systems combined present a range of techniques that enable MAPPA to compile risk assessment information and strategies for risk management, including any breaches or failures:

- *Soft surveillance* is located within the exchange between MAPPA members and relies on a range of information sharing techniques including wide access to probation, police and social work records and an extension of the use of psychiatric and medical records. Such formal information, underpinned by joint information sharing protocols and agreements, is supplemented by a reliance on observations and anecdotal 'stories' and police intelligence networks.

- *Technologies of surveillance* are evident throughout the MAPPA process with electronic risk assessment tools (e-OASys), databases for the monitoring of MAPPA cases, ViSOR (see Probation Circular 40/2006), and review systems based on electronically recorded panel minutes. The community protection measures also comprise most risk management plans, with technological solutions provided to enforce curfews, restrictions and management of spaces (such as the tagging of offenders).

Both methods demonstrate covert forms of surveillance with the offender involvement severely restricted and an emphasis on the professional and technological management of risk. Offenders are not significantly involved in the process of risk management planning (apart from one example of a MAPPA that involves offenders in panel meetings; Mikulski, 2004).

The construction of the offender, the problem with perceptions and fears associated with sex offenders, together with the availability of technology have all led to a creeping growth of the surveillance system, with seemingly little opposition to such measures. Surveillance has also been extended to violent offenders (see the 2003 CJA).

Risk management and regulation

Although given statutory responsibility and some degree of public accountability through annual reports, MAPPA are characterised by a lack of regulation and transparency (Kemshall et al, 2005). Lay involvement is limited to two advisors on Strategic Management Boards (some distance from the daily operational decision making of MAPPA), and while there is accountability for performance to the Home Office Public Protection and Licence Unit, this does not constitute a regulatory and governance system to ensure that risk management remains ethical, just, fair and proportionate. This lack of regulation in effect allows for a creeping growth in surveillance and justification of measures on a 'case by case' basis that results in a general application to groups of offenders (what is justified for one paedophile becomes justified for all).

Risk management is also increasingly about exclusionary techniques, despite some limited rhetoric to the contrary. The overriding prioritisation is one of public protection, with offender rehabilitation often seen as only a potential supplementary aim (Wood and Kemshall,

2007). Surveillance keeps offenders 'in place', usually at the margins, and rarely fulfils any integrative function. Community protection begins to take on hallmarks of custody in the community, with constraints, restrictions, and intensive management of offender time and space (for example, by curfews and exclusion zones).

Conclusion

The stigmatisation and public loathing of sex offenders (described by Jenny Kitzinger, 1999, as the 'ultimate neighbour from hell') is used to justify both the community containment of sex offenders and the erosion of their rights. This is extending to other high-risk offenders, for example violent offenders. Human rights and ethical considerations are more easily disregarded when the offender group concerned is among the most loathsome and the most feared. Public perceptions of sex offenders and fear of the 'Monsters in our Midst' (Channel Four, 1998) have played a significant role in the development of policy and legislation in this area (see Thomas, 2001, 2005; Kitzinger, 2004, for a full review). It has also left this offender group without natural allies or advocates – the offending is itself taboo, and there is the fear of tainting oneself by association. Risks have largely justified the erosion of rights, and the vulnerability of potential victims (usually children) has also outweighed any ethical questioning of risk management plans.

However, current judicial reviews and challenges under the ECHR ensure that some tension remains in the system between public protection and individual rights. Within this, there is considerable evidence that practitioners attempt to operate according to the available guidance, and are at pains to ensure appropriate audit trails and a degree of transparency for their decisions. There is also evidence of 'best practice' initiatives that attempt to promote individual reintegration and rehabilitation while ensuring public safety. Offenders themselves understand and largely respond positively to such approaches. The issue for them is not one of an abstract right, but how they are actually treated and what positive outcomes for them are actually achieved by MAPPA.

Note
[1] Thanks are extended to those colleagues who worked with us on the MAPPA evaluation studies cited. However, the views expressed here do not necessarily represent the views of colleagues or report co-authors and are entirely the responsibility of the chapter authors.

References

BBC Online (2007) *Britons' Foreign Crimes 'Ignored'*, http://news.bbc. co.uk/1/hi/uk/6239727.stm

Bichard, Sir Michael (2004) *The Bichard Inquiry Report*, London: The Stationery Office.

Channel Four (1998) *Monsters in our Midst: Community Perceptions of Sex Offenders*, 8 January.

Connelly, C. and Williamson, S. (2000) *Review of the Research Literature on Serious Violent and Sexual Offenders*, Crime and Criminal Justice Research Findings No. 46, Edinburgh: Scottish Executive Central Research Unit.

Elbogen, E.B., Patry, M. and Scalora, M.J. (2003) 'The impact of community notification laws on sex offender attitudes', *International Journal of Law and Psychiatry*, vol 26, no 2, pp 207-19.

HMIP (Her Majesty's Inspectorate of Probation) (2006a) *An Independent Review of a Serious Further Offence Case: Damien Hanson and Elliot White*, London: HMIP.

HMIP (2006b) *An Independent Review of a Serious Further Offence Case: Anthony Rice*, London: HMIP.

Home Office (2004) *MAPPA Guidance*, London: Home Office.

Home Office (2006a) *Rebalancing the Criminal Justice System in Favour of the Law Abiding Majority: Cutting Crime, Reducing Reoffending and Protecting the Public*, London: Home Office.

Home Office (2006b) *The Home Secretary's Five Year Strategy for Protecting the Public and Reducing Reoffending*, Announced 9 February, London: Home Office.

Kemshall, H. (2001) *Risk Assessment and Management of Known Sexual and Violent Offenders: A Review of Current Issues*, Police Research Series 140, London: Home Office.

Kemshall, H. (2003) *Understanding Risk in Criminal Justice*, Buckingham: Open University Press.

Kemshall, H., Wood, J., Mackenzie, G., Bailey, R. and Yates, J. (2005) *Strengthening Multi-Agency Public Protection Arrangements (MAPPA)*, London: Home Office.

Kitzinger, J. (1999) 'The ultimate neighbour from hell: media framing of paedophiles', in B. Franklin (ed) *Social Policy, Media and Misrepresentation*, London: Routledge.

Kitzinger, J. (2004) *Framing Abuse: Media Influence and Public Understanding of Sexual Violence against Children*, London: Pluto Press.

Lovell, E. (2001) *Megan's Law: Does it Protect Children? A Review of the Evidence on the Impact of Community Notification as Legislated for through Megan's Law in the United States: Recommendations for Policy Makers in the United Kingdom*, London: NSPCC.

Maguire, M., Kemshall, H., Noaks, L. and Wincup, E. (2001) *Risk Management of Sexual and Violent Offenders: The Work of Public Protection Panels*, Police Research Series 139, London: Home Office.

Mikulski, A. (2004) 'Managing the unmanageable: dangerous offenders and the MAPPA process', Paper presented to the British Society of Criminology Conference, Portsmouth, 8 July.

Nash, M. (2006) *Public Protection and the Criminal Justice Process*, Oxford: Oxford University Press.

Petrunik, M. (2003) 'The hare and the tortoise: dangerous and sex offender policy in the United States and Canada', *Canadian Journal of Criminology and Criminal Justice*, vol 45, no 1, pp 43-72.

Probation Circular 40/2006, *ViSOR implementation*, London: National Probation Service.

Royal College of Psychiatrists (2004) *Psychiatrists and Multi-Agency Public Protection Arrangements*, www.rcpsych.ac.uk/members/membership/public_protection.htm

Thomas, T. (2001) 'Sex offenders, the Home Office and the Sunday papers', *Journal of Social Welfare and Family Law*, vol 23, no 1, pp 103-8.

Thomas, T. (2003) 'Sex offender community notification: experiences from America', *Howard Journal of Criminal Justice*, vol 42, no 3, pp 217-28.

Thomas, T. (2005) *Sex Crime: Sex Offending and Society* (2nd edition), Cullompton: Willan.

Wood, J. and Kemshall, H., with Maguire, M., Hudson, K. and Mackenzie, G. (2007) *The Operation and Experience of Multi-Agency Public Protection Arrangements*, London: Home Office.

SEVEN

The right to information in practice: adoption records, confidentiality and secrecy

Gary Clapton

As I was growing up, my parents rarely mentioned my adoption. It didn't interfere with our life together. They always introduced me as 'our daughter,' rather than 'our adopted daughter'. I was born in the days when adoption agencies screened genealogy of birth and adoptive families to choose people with similar characteristics. My Dad and I are both tall with medium brown hair and blue-green eyes. I looked like I belonged. It was easy to keep my secret. I only told a handful of people.

My Dad confided that there was a paper he would give me when I turned 21. I tried to say it didn't matter. But on my 21st birthday, I waited. Dad drew a manila envelope from a locked file in his study ... he teased, 'Do you think you're tough enough to take this?' (Campbell, 2003)

Introduction

This chapter concerns adoption and secrecy. It is about the people involved in adoptions. The chapter is designed to open up debate. The discussion draws from the author's research (Clapton, 2003, 2006) and 10 years' experience as an adoption counsellor, and also from discussions with the staff of Birthlink, an after-adoption service run by Scottish-based adoption agency Family Care.

Reference is very often made to the 'adoption triad': the adopted person, the adoptive parents and the birth parents. All too often the fourth party directly involved in adoption – the social worker – is omitted. Here the importance of this fourth person in adoption is acknowledged. The discussion concentrates on the adoptions of the 1950s, 1960s and 1970s.

As adults, many of those who were adopted as babies in the 'non-relative' adoptions from this period seek information to help them make sense of their origins, medical histories and identities. In keeping with a rise of interest in genealogical information and family history, there has been a growth in demand for access to the information held by adoption agencies concerning the circumstances of adopted people's conception, birth and adoption and the background and motivations of their birth parents. This search involves negotiating with the gatekeepers of this information – social workers and adoption agency record holders. As will be seen, accessing information in adoption is neither straightforward nor painless. It is far from the simple open-access exercise that may be imagined.

Adoption and secrecy: 'a blank and impenetrable wall between the identities of natural and adopting parents'

This quotation comes from a 1957 book of advice to adoptive parents cited by Samuels (2001, p 399). It has been argued that secrecy and confidentiality have been part of the legal institution of adoption from its inception (Haimes and Timms, 1985). Adoption is arguably the most secret of all processes involving a child. It is the process by which children cease to be the legal sons or daughters of their birth parents and become, instead, the children of adoptive parents. The records of that first life are then substituted by another and locked up, often only to be partially accessed, and under certain conditions. Should the child grow up and wish to know something about his (or her) origins, then he will discover that there are few other circumstances in which adults have such difficulty in accessing information about themselves, such as their medical history, the circumstances of their birth and details of their parentage. Adoption is where the need for confidentiality and secrecy meet. There are three parts to this process.

First, when a child leaves his birth family for an adoptive family, his name is changed officially, his original birth certificate is annotated 'adopted' and an Adoption Certificate is issued as a replacement. This certificate carries the date of the adoption order and the details of the court that approved this together with the child's new name and date of birth. An abbreviated version of the Adoption Certificate carrying only name and date of birth is regularly issued, thus avoiding reference to the adoption when simple proof of identity is required. In Scotland, unlike England, the register containing details of Adoption Certificates is not available to the public. In both Scotland and England, there is no public means to cross-check the register of births with the register of adoptions (Rushbrooke, 2001). Notwithstanding these restrictions there have never been any conditions placed on adopted people who wish to access their birth certificates in Scotland. Someone adopted before 1975 in England and Wales must have an interview with a designated counsellor before being entitled to receive a copy of their original birth certificate. Requirements such as this and the Scottish practice of maintaining a private Register of Adoptions create an air of taboo around a basic building block of identity, one's birth certificate.

Second, court records relating to the adoption are sealed. These records are entitled Court Process and only the adopted adult may see these. Court Process records are probably the least known of adoption records, yet they contain the legal papers relating to the adoption and the signature of the person who relinquishes the child for adoption, who is usually the birth mother. In Scotland, the right to view Court Process is untrammelled; however, someone adopted through an English court must apply to the court for permission to see the records. For an older adult, unwrapping the official government-issue envelope tied with string and wax-sealed, written in the copperplate of a long-dead clerk to the court, is a highly charged emotional experience representing the physical opening of a secret meant to be forever buried.

Third, if an adoption agency is involved the files are locked away. In nearly half of the adoptions in the period in question, there was no adoption agency involved and therefore there are no adoption files or social workers' records. In such cases, the adoption may have been initiated by a general practitioner or church minister and the investigatory aspect undertaken by an appointee of the court. Where an agency was involved files may contain records of interviews with the birth mother and possibly also her parents. These can range from one page to several typed sheets detailing a sequence of office interviews at which the painful decision to relinquish is arrived at. Compounding the sense of secrecy, or at least inaccessibility, is the fact that many of these agencies have either closed or been renamed or the records have been destroyed, as is the case with the files of one 'prolific' Scottish adoption organisation, the National Vigilance Society (Glasgow branch).

Why secrecy?

The rationale for the secrecy surrounding adoptions was the notion that a 'veil of secrecy' was vital for the well-being of all concerned. In her analysis of adoption policy and practice in the US in the 1950s and 1960s – which are akin to that of the same period in the UK (see Sants, 1964) – Samuels (2001) writes of a 'universal regime of secrecy' (p 370) with the adoptive child's origins 'cloaked in secrecy' (p 385). Such policy and practice was justified on three main grounds. First, adoptive parents would be protected from any distress associated with notions of raising an illegitimate child – the child was to be raised 'as if' born to them; this also helped avoid any awkward discussion about infertility. Agencies went to great lengths to achieve a match of physical characteristics and presumed intellectual ability in order to make the 'as if born to' notion as tenable as possible (Kellmer-Pringle, 1972). Second, an adoption that was 'closed' would help adopted children be raised without the stigma of 'bad blood' (Samuels, 2001, p 385). An adoption is described as 'closed' here in contrast to the later move towards openness in adoption, which is marked by efforts to have contact between birth families, adopted children and adoptive families prior to, during and after the adoption. Third, unmarried mothers would be shielded from societal opprobrium (Van Bueren, 1995). As much help as possible was rendered to ensure that the birth could take place away from the mother's home surroundings (Petrie, 1998).

However, it was the needs of the adoptive family that were paramount in the rationale for closed adoptions. In the words of the then Irish Minister for Justice in a discussion of the Irish Adoption Bill in 1974:

> It is basic to our adoption code that the adopted child becomes the child of the adoptive parents in everything except the natural blood. *It would be contrary to that principle if we allowed to be introduced into that relationship curiosity or questions concerning the natural ancestry of the child.* We want to ensure that the family together with the adopted child becomes as far as possible a natural family, bonded in terms of natural love as the Minister for Posts and Telegraphs said. We want to achieve that aim and it would be going against that if we were to facilitate information regarding the ancestry of the adopted child to be given to him. So far as possible we want to make him the child of the adoptive parents and this is the reason for having our code of adoption

as is, preserving the secrecy of his origin from the child. (Minister for Justice, Mr Cooney, *Dáil Eireann*, vol 273, 5 June 1974; emphasis added)

It can be seen that well into the 1970s, it was felt that in order to join and thrive in an adoptive family, all mention of and references to the child's family by birth ought to be kept hidden or at least unmentioned. Adoptive parents were assured that '[i]nstances of extreme curiosity and concern almost never happen' (Le Shan, 1958).

   The requirement that an adopted child be legally treated 'as if born to' remains in the UK today (2002 Adoption and Children Act, section 67). However, as can be seen, adoption policy and practice have tended to conflate this legal requirement with the myth that the adoptive family was not different from birth families. The child would be considered, treated and raised to all intents and purposes as if they were indeed the parents by blood (Kirk, 1964; Samuels, 2001) and that the birth parents had somehow been cancelled out by the adoptive parents. 'You have no right to any information whatsoever. You were adopted legally.... You had no other parents' (adoption lawyer quoted in Fisher, 1973, p 84). It follows that the child's origins had something of the forbidden about them. This outlook had (and has) major implications should adopted children raise the matter or discover that their adoptive status had been kept from them.

Discovering the shoebox at the bottom of the wardrobe

Should a youngster ever raise the question, (Who are my birth-parents?) it is important, of course, to make it very clear that a search is unrealistic and can lead to unhappiness and disillusionment. (*You and Your Adopted Child*, Public Affairs Pamphlet, New York, 1958)

At almost the same time that the Irish Minister for Justice was maintaining the need for secrecy, research undertaken by John Triseliotis (1973) disproved the notion that curiosity about one's origins was a sign of pathology or poor adoptive family upbringing. Yet the belief that there was something wrong with an adopted person who became curious about his (or her) origins was powerful. Samuels (2001) cites examples of the prevailing outlook in the 1960s and 1970s and quotes one leading psychiatrist as saying:

> Occasionally we see tragically pathological distortions
> ... very disturbed young people who ... develop an all-
> consuming, obsessing need to locate their biological parents
> who in fantasy, or even delusion, have become the idealized
> good parents in contrast to the adoptive 'bad' parents with
> whom they are usually no longer in contact. (Bernard,
> quoted in Samuels, 2001, pp 409-10)

Drawing on research into adoption agency practice, Samuels (2001, p 410) quotes from one agency's manual that characterised a searching adopted adult as 'a person who has had many unhappy past experiences and ... is so intent upon finding the natural parent that he is not able to consider his request in a realistic or rational way'. The manual advised caseworkers to discourage the search and then, if necessary, to refer the person for psychological treatment. Betty Lifton, a prominent campaigning adopted person, recounts being told by a psychiatrist when she was in the early stages of seeking information about her origins that 'your need to look for your mother is neurotic' (quoted in Samuels, 2001, p 403).

Despite the findings of Triseliotis and many other researchers since (Brodzinsky and Schechter, 1990), a powerful belief remains in the damage that can be caused by the release of information relating to an adopted person's origin and adoption. This is never clearer than in the continuing practice in the US whereby most states adhere to the 'sealed record' philosophy – no birth family information is available to the adopted adult, not even the original birth certificate (Baer, 2004). This is not to say that practice in the UK is now free from such an outlook. Although the practice of openness has grown over the past 20 years, the fact is that many adults who approach after-adoption services today were born in the 1960s and 1970s (and before) and have grown up within a culture of secrecy surrounding their adoption (Triseliotis et al, 1997; Rushbrooke, 2001; Davies, 2003; Elliot, 2005).

In the literature and the accounts of adopted people there are many incidents of surprise and shock caused by hearing about their adoption from school playground taunts, parental outbursts during adolescence and, in extreme cases, on finding their adoption papers in a shoebox in the bottom of a wardrobe when clearing out the parental home after the last living adoptive parent had died (*Secrets and Lies*, 1996, dir. Mike Leigh; Iredale, 1997; TALKAdoption, 1999). If a message from adoptive parents was one either tinged with shame ('it was mentioned once, then dropped despite my best efforts to raise it again') or secrecy ('I only found out when I had to apply for a passport in my own right'), then it is no wonder that the adopted adult may approach the question of information with some ambivalence, to say the least (McWhinnie, 1984). Van Bueren (1995, p 39) provides a historical example where even ambivalence would have been a dangerous luxury:

> Under the code of laws promulgated by Hammurabi, King of Babylon 2285-2242 BC, adoptees risked having their tongues cut out if they stated openly that they had not been born to their adopted parents and could be blinded if they attempted to search for their biological parents.

If information has not been entirely forthcoming, then actively seeking it becomes a matter fraught with difficulties.

First steps, first hurdles

It is now well established that adopted people's curiosity about their origins is valid, necessary and to be encouraged (Triseliotis, 1973; Brodzinsky and Schechter, 1990; Grotevant, 1997; Triseliotis et al, 1997). In a study of the motivations of 472 adopted people, Howe et al (2001, p 346) found that:

> the most common reasons given for searching for a birth relative included such remarks as 'getting information about me to help complete the jigsaw' and 'the need to know more about myself and make the picture whole'.

According to Neil (2000, p 303):

> It is important for adopted people to know not only the details of their biological heritage, but to explore the question of *why* they were adopted. This entails understanding the issues that led to the adoption, including the circumstances of the birthparents and the actions of social workers and agencies.

Neil (2000, p 304) goes on to state that 'the need to know the truth is compelling'.

In addition to such motivation that has, arguably, always been present in adopted people, in keeping with today's greater interest in and awareness of the importance of genealogical information, more adopted adults than before feel that they ought to have greater access to information surrounding their adoption and family of origin (Rushbrooke, 2001; Trinder et al, 2004; Triseliotis et al, 2005). Based on their research with 74 adopted adults, Trinder et al (2004) suggest that now something like 50% of adopted people will seek information. Indeed, one researcher has gone as far to say that 'we should perhaps explore why some adoptees do not search, rather than see it as a minority activity' (Selman, 1999). Yet this growing number of adopted people must negotiate both external and inner hurdles to achieve their aspiration.

Externally, there is a lack of knowledge regarding the variety and widespread nature of the information that may be available in respect of their adoption and origins: 'the adopted person who really wishes to discover his genetic history will require persistence and tenacity as well as skills of detection' (Freeman, 1996, p 278). Before even seeing anything to do with his (or her) early life, an adopted person may have expended considerable effort in discovering where to go, what exists and who to ask (Haimes, 1988). Schechter and Bertocci (1990, p 62) talk of 'a nearly impenetrable iron curtain between herself and her genealogical background'. Once accessed, information that Haimes (1988, p 58) has described as 'institutionally hidden', may be conflicting, inaccurate, or both. All of this makes the accessing of officially held information on adoption a highly emotionally charged and exhausting journey. The legal and policy variations across the UK and lack of practitioner knowledge in how to access legally available records such as birth certificates and Court Process, and adopted people's difficulties in obtaining information regarding their origins would make the subject of another chapter.

Within the adopted person, the legacy of secrecy may constitute an injunction against seeking out information:

> Although more liberal attitudes were more prevalent during the 1960s, the vast majority of the adoptees ... would have been brought up under the 'new start' philosophy that held that adoptees would never need their birth records. In some cases, perhaps many cases, this view of adoption would have been assimilated at an unconscious level without ever having been formally discussed. For many adoptees in this group, therefore, the process of applying for their birth records will have involved a fundamental change in how they thought about their identity. (Rushbrooke, 2001, p 30)

In Iredale's (1997) accounts of adopted people's meetings with their birth relatives, one adopted person feared asking her parents for information: 'I was scared of upsetting the apple cart by broaching the subject' (p 151); for another, raising the matter was at the least a 'guessing game' (p 152). It seems, then, that the development of the fortitude often required to chase down records depends first of all on winning the struggle to be allowed to grow up.

Secrecy in adoption and the infantilisation of adopted people

It is not uncommon for adopted adults to be treated as an adopted child; as if somehow the act of adoption froze them in a permanently infantile state (Grimm, 1997; Robinson, 2005, p 12). In their discussion of the similarities between the positions of adopted people and those who have been conceived by artificial insemination Blyth et al (2001, p 301) remark:

> Although real comparison is made difficult by varying legislative and regulatory arrangements in different countries, a pervasive theme is that both adopted people and donor offspring are liable to be ascribed the status of children even when they reach legal adulthood. Their dependence on the state and their own parents for information about their origins further emphasizes the significance of power and information control in socially created families.

An example of how institutional practice infantilises adopted adults is that when they seek to gain access to information about their roots they must receive services from children's services teams as if still 'children' and objects of decision making.

Feelings of powerlessness are seen as being rooted in the adoption process itself. After-adoption counsellors have often heard the phrases 'no one asked me' and 'I was moved around like an unwanted parcel'. Modell (1994, p 151) draws attention to such feelings among adopted people when she notes that, for an adopted adult, '[b]eing defined as less than adult and not in control of one's own life course was not unique to searching adoptees, but it was certainly part of their experience'. This might account for the descriptions of 'angry', 'difficult' and having a 'chip on their shoulder' made about adopted people by those who have not been adopted. Few studies have explored the interpersonal dynamics involved in the adopted person's efforts to navigate between record holders and piece together information. It may be no exaggeration to say that as much energy may be spent in this struggle – in essence, to be allowed to mature – as can be devoted to tracking down the information.

Assuming, then, that the adopted adult has learnt to live with familial and societal pressures to infantilise him, the next step is the search for the documents. This journey is rendered in a linear fashion here but in practice it involves stops and starts, regressions and recoveries.

Opening Pandora's Box: accessing adoption agency records

The case files – the unofficial, non-public records held by adoption agencies – are a much less regulated area of adoption practice. For the many 'private' adoptions that have taken place there are next to no papers other than the original birth certificate and Court Process. An adoption may be arranged by an adoption society or a local authority; before 1984, when it became illegal, an adoption may have been organised by an individual such as a solicitor, doctor or priest acting in a private capacity. Records in the latter type of adoption, other than those that were legally necessary, are generally absent. However, where an adoption agency was involved, there is often a case file. These can vary in length from one sheet to many pages of detailed entries made by social workers at the centre of the official part of the adoption process. Such UK records must be kept for 75 years. Access to the information in these varies (Rushbrooke, 2001), making for a 'postcode lottery', for the simple reason that there is no right of adopted adults to see adoption case records. Neither is there any requirement for the sharing of any information contained in such papers. In the phrase on Glasgow City Council's web page, 'the disclosure of information is at the discretion of the agency' (www.glasgow.gov.uk/en/Residents/Care_Support/Families_Children/Adoption_Fostering/OriginSearch/).

While it may be that practice among adoption record holders now generally tends towards access, the *type* and *extent* of access varies in a complex and confusing mixture of vagueness as to what is 'allowed', efforts to protect historical policies and practices, and notions of third party protection. Access to records can range from the provision of an edited version through to the complete sharing of the contents of the file. Information may be made available in the form of a transcript of selected key points, or solely via a conversation with a social worker who has accessed the information, or as a read-through of a microfiche of all or an edited part of the file. In the most liberal instances it comprises the provision of photocopies of the full records. In some cases sharing of the material is only partial and agencies have been known to divulge only the first name of a birth father on the grounds that although named as the father by the birth mother, there is nothing to prove this. This prejudices his interest since he is denied the opportunity to prove or disprove whether he is the father. In other instances, social workers may actively suppress what they consider to be disturbing information. In her discussion of the content of adoption files and social workers' dilemmas in sharing information, Gannon (2005, p 61) quotes workers as saying that 'they would write a summary of certain events in the child's life if they felt the information would be particularly painful to receive'. This form of censorship, albeit well meaning, perpetuates secrecy and double standards. What if two adopted adults approach an agency for information from their records and one gets a summary while the other gets the full set of photocopies? What might each conclude if they were to compare these experiences? That in the latter's case there was nothing to hide, whereas in the former person's records ... what?

In another case, one worker in Gannon's study abbreviates the information not so much out of expurgation but because the style of the written record seems to jar: 'I might summarise and explain that I've written this because I don't like the way it was written' (quoted in Gannon, 2005, p 61). Elsewhere, however, another respondent believes that 'the truth is of more benefit' (2005, p 62). Gannon observes that all eight of her respondents struggled with the decision 'of what, how much and when to tell' (2005, p 62). The views and practices of the social workers in Gannon's study go to the heart of the matter. This is the issue of power and powerlessness in adoption. Anyone working in adoption and providing a service should understand this and the impact of their judgement. They may, of course, already do so if they are a birth parent or an adopted person.

Dismantling secrecy

In the last 23 years, therefore, we have witnessed an unprecedented event amongst the adopted population that was completely unexpected, that has affected a relatively large number of people, that is far from complete and that, in terms of the underlying psychological motives of those involved, is still a long way from being fully understood. (Rushbrooke, 2001, p 31)

The central argument of this chapter is: good practice in adoption means dismantling secrecy. Remember that adopted people may have been treated like children all their lives in relation to the 'secret' of their origins. The 60-year-old woman sitting opposite has a reason to be angry, unpredictable or tearful. Adopted people need the same access to their histories that everyone else enjoys. Censorship and secrecy breed suspicion. Adopted persons who finally get within physical reach of their records (their life) may very well have undergone a mentally and physically taxing journey to finally arrive where they have needed to be for years. Treat adopted people as the adults they are – not the infants they once were. Half-truths and evasions have been the stuff of much of their lives. To continue to treat adopted people as children is to perpetuate an injustice.

In an unpublished court decision later reversed by the South Carolina Supreme Court, the judge wrote:

> The law must be constant with life. It cannot and should not ignore broad historical currents of history. Mankind is possessed of no greater urge than to try to understand the age-old questions: 'Who am I?' 'Why am I?' Even now the sands and ashes of the continents are being sifted where we made our first steps as man. Religions of mankind often include ancestor worship in one way or another. For many, the future is blind without a sight of the past. Those emotions and anxieties that generate our thirst to know the past are not superficial and whimsical. They are real and they are 'good cause' under the law of man and God. (Justice Bradey, 1979)

Or put more simply: 'no person should be cut off from his origins' (Triseliotis, 1984).

What could be circumstances under which someone ought not to read their adoption records? To ask this is to run the risk of diluting the main thrust of this chapter, which calls for an end to the protectionism that exists within adoption practice. Sometimes the stick needs to be bent in the opposite direction. However, in the interests of balance, what can be said?

All sorts of reasons for denying access may be put and there is not space here to detail them, but they can include protection of the sensibilities of birth mothers, the safeguarding of promises of anonymity to adoptive parents, and an unwillingness to open up the historically poor practices of social workers and adoption agencies or to reveal confidentially supplied information from other professionals named in the files. However, the agency record holder currently remains, so to speak, judge and jury when it comes to granting or denying a case for access to adoption records. This review of past and developing practices suggests that in the event of a dispute over access, the case ought to be heard by a higher or independent body and the final decision ought not to remain with social workers and adoption record holders.

Cases concerning access to adoption records have already come before the courts. In 1999 the Nugent Care Society refused to reveal information from its adoption case files on Linda Gunn-Russo, who was adopted in 1948. Aided by Liberty, the civil rights campaigning organisation, Gunn-Russo took her case to law and won. The case was heard in the Administrative Court in May 2001. Mr Justice Scott Baker ruled that the Society had to reconsider its position. He held that the Society's policy on disclosure was too rigid 'in the light of present day circumstances' and went on to say:

> Most reasonable people would not I think feel that after half a century disclosure would be likely to impair public confidence in the integrity of the system. After all a great many public records are now disclosed after thirty years. (Neutral Citation Number: [2001] EWHC Admin 566)

After the judgment, Gunn-Russo said: 'Hopefully it'll open files up for people all over the country. We won't have to sit back and take no for an answer when we ask about our parents and our early lives. It's about our personal identification' (Liberty, Press Release, 20 July 2001).

The Gunn-Russo judgment is a milestone in adopted people's struggle to obtain what they need from their case files. It echoes the judgment in the case of Graham Gaskin, who grew up in local authority care in Liverpool and was later refused access to his files. Gaskin appealed to the European Court of Human Rights in Strasbourg. The Court decided in 1989 that Gaskin's Article 8 right to have his private and family life respected by the state had been breached by the UK government. The Court also decided that people in Gaskin's position, who had been in public care as children, should not in principle be obstructed from accessing their care records (Gaskin, 2005).

The advantage of going to law is that an adopted person would have an advocate to argue the case for access to his (or her) origins. This, of course, raises the question of cost to the adopted person. Should the cost not be borne by the adoption record holder as a demonstration of goodwill? This might help focus official minds on whether denial of access is really based on risk to rights or is just a matter of established ideology, policy or practice. An alternative to a legal process could be the establishment of independent review panels made up of adopted people, birth parents, adoptive parents and an agency representative.

What of those whose capacity to understand may be impaired, such as some people with severe learning disabilities? People in such circumstances ought to have the same right to access as anyone else. How they, and their families, are supported to make sense of the consequent information is a professional support task that may be undertaken by a dedicated advocate or mentor working alongside them. Because, again, as for people without disabilities, the question of origins is not only one for adopted persons themselves; it is also a vital building block in identity formation for the children of adopted people.

Conclusion

In *Secrets*, Bok (1989, p 7) writes that 'the link between secrecy and deceit is so strong in the minds of some that they mistakenly take all secrecy to be deceptive'. This chapter has argued that often the reality for adopted adults has been that deceit and secrecy are indistinguishable, and that the potent mix of attitudes and the adoption policy and practices described infantilises them – and in some cases infuriates. Adopted people have often been denied agency, the opportunity to be masters of their own lives. Secrecy is part of the problem and definitely not part of the solution.

It follows, then, that professionals ought to do everything within their power to ensure that the 'good cause' referred to by Justice Bradey is understood and not denied. The challenge for professionals is how to listen and help adopted adults – and not become another obstacle in what is already a difficult enough journey towards truth.

References

Baer, J. (2004) *Growing in the Dark: Adoption Secrecy and its Consequences*, California, CA: Xlibris Corporation.

Blyth, E., Crawshaw, M., Haase, J. and Speirs, J. (2001) 'The implications of adoption for donor offspring following donor-assisted conception', *Child & Family Social Work*, vol 6, no 4, pp 295-304.

Bok, S. (1989) *Secrets: On the Ethics of Concealment and Revelation*, New York: Vintage.

Bradey, Justice (1979) in *Bradey v Children's Bureau*, S.C. Ct. Com. Pl., 9 April 1979, quoted in Harrington, J. (1980) 'The courts contend with sealed adoption records', *Public Welfare*, pp 29-43.

Brodzinsky, D. and Schechter, M. (eds) (1990) *The Psychology of Adoption*, Oxford: Oxford University Press.

Campbell, C. (2003) 'Southern blood, western roots', *Znine*, www.uta.edu/english/znines03/cf3.htm

Clapton, G. (2003) *Relatively Unknown: A Year in the Life of the Adoption Contact Register for Scotland*, Edinburgh: Family Care.

Clapton, G. (2006) 'Mediated contact: reflections on a piece of after-adoption intermediary practice', *Adoption and Fostering*, vol 30, no 4, pp 53-63.

Davies, H. (2003) *Relative Strangers: A History of Adoption and a Tale of Triplets*, London: Little, Brown.

Elliott, S. (2005) *Love Child: A Memoir of Adoption, Loss And Love*, London: Vermillion.

Fisher, F. (1973) *The Search for Anna Fisher*, New York: Fawcett Crest Books.

Freeman, M. (1996) 'The new birth right? Identity and the child of the reproduction revolution', *International Journal of Children's Rights*, vol 4, pp 273-97.

Gannon, J. (2005) 'Holding and sharing memories: the significance of social work recording for birth record counselling', *Adoption and Fostering*, vol 29, no 4, pp 57-67.

Gaskin, G. (2005) *A Boy Called Graham*, London: Blake Publishing.

Grimm, S. (1997) 'Why contact vetoes are not an acceptable compromise', *Bastard Quarterly*, Spring, Bastard Nation.

Grotevant, H. (1997) 'Coming to terms with adoption: the construction of identity from adolescence into adulthood', *Adoption Quarterly*, vol 1, pp 3-27.

Haimes, E. (1988) 'Secrecy: what can artificial reproduction learn from adoption?', *International Journal of Law and the Family*, vol 2, pp 46-61.

Haimes, E. and Timms, N. (1985) *Adoption, Identity and Social Policy: The Search for Distant Relatives*, Aldershot: Gower.

Howe, D., Shemmings, D. and Feast, J. (2001) 'Age at placement and adult adopted people's experience of being adopted', *Child & Family Social Work*, vol 6, no 4, pp 337-49.

Iredale, S. (1997) *Reunions: True Stories of Adoptees' Meetings with their Natural Parents*, London: The Stationery Office.

Kellmer-Pringle, M. (1972) 'A place of one's own', in J. Seglow, M. Kellmer-Pringle and P. Wedge (eds) *Growing Up Adopted*, London: National Foundation for Education Research, pp 163-82.

Kirk, H. (1964) *Shared Fate: A Theory of Adoption and Mental Health*, New York: Free Press.

Le Shan, E. (1958) *You and Your Adopted Child*, Public Affairs Pamphlet No. 274, New York: Public Affairs Committee.

McWhinnie, A. (1984) 'Annex: The case for greater openness concerning AID', in British Agencies for Adoption and Fostering (ed) *AID and After*, London: BAAF.

Modell, J. (1994) *Kinship with Strangers: Adoption and Interpretations of Kinship in American Culture*, Berkeley, CA: University of California Press.

Neil, E. (2000) 'The reasons why young children are placed for adoption: findings from a recently placed sample and a discussion of implications for subsequent identity development', *Child & Family Social Work*, vol 5, no 4, pp 303–16.

ONS (Office for National Statistics) (2006) *Marriage, Divorce and Adoption Statistics: Review of the Registrar General on Marriages and Divorces in 2003, and adoptions in 2004, in England and Wales*, London: Palgrave Macmillan.

Petrie, A. (1998) *Gone to an Aunt's: Remembering Canada's Homes for Unwed Mothers*, Toronto: McClelland and Stewart.

Robinson, E. (2005) *Natural Parents News*, Spring, Natural Parents Network.

Rushbrooke, R. (2001) 'The proportion of adoptees who have received their birth records in England and Wales', *Population Trends*, no 104, London: Office for National Statist ics, pp 26–34.

Samuels, E. (2001) 'The idea of adoption: an inquiry into the history of adult adoptee access to birth records', *Rutgers Law Review*, Winter, pp 367–437.

Sants, H. (1964) 'Genealogical bewilderment in children with substitute parents', *British Journal of Medical Psychology*, vol 37, pp 133–41.

Schechter, D. and Bertocci, D. (1990) 'The meaning of the search', in D. Brodzinsky and D. Schechter (eds) *The Psychology of Adoption*, Oxford: Oxford University Press, pp 62–92.

Selman, P. (1999) 'In search of origins: estimating life time take-up of access to birth records in England & Wales', Poster Presentation at the International Conference on Adoption Research, Minneapolis, 10–15 August.

TALKAdoption (1999) 'Many young people do not know that they are adopted – findings from national helpline', Press Release, 29 November, Manchester: TALKAdoption.

Trinder, E., Feast, J. and Howe, D. (2004) *The Adoption Reunion Handbook*, Chichester: John Wiley.

Triseliotis, J. (1973) *In Search of Origins: The Experiences of Adopted People*, London: Routledge & Kegan Paul.

Triseliotis, J. (1984) 'Obtaining birth certificates', in P. Bean (ed) *Adoption*, London: Tavistock.

Triseliotis, J., Feast, J. and Kyle, F. (2005) *The Adoption Triangle Revisited: A Study of Adoption, Search and Reunion Experiences*, London: BAAF.

Triseliotis, J., Shireman, J. and Hundleby, M. (1997) *Adoption: Theory, Policy and Practice*, London: Cassell.

Van Bueren, G. (1995) 'Children's access to adoption records – state discretion or an enforceable international right?', *The Modern Law Review*, vol 58, no 1, pp 37-53.

Part Three
Working together

EIGHT

Confidentiality and information sharing in child protection

Janice McGhee

Introduction

The direction of UK and Scottish government policy towards the promotion of 'joint working' between agencies and professionals and the advent of multidisciplinary teams has made information sharing more central to effective practice and service delivery. Tensions can arise, however, between differing professional guidelines (Crichton, 2001). In child welfare the importance of interagency cooperation and information sharing to protect children at risk of abuse and neglect is longstanding and is reflected in government guidance and interagency protocols and procedure including multiagency case conferences (Scottish Office, 1998; Scottish Executive, 2003; DfES, 2006a). The UK child protection system developed from the mid-1970s following the report of the inquiry into the death of Maria Colwell (DHSS, 1974) and emphasises investigation and surveillance combined with extensive procedural guidance, including that on sharing information (Waterhouse and McGhee, 2002). Effective practice to assess risk in relation to a child is seen as dependent on interagency cooperation and information sharing (Hallett and Birchall, 1992; DH, 1995); nevertheless, tensions do arise in practice.

It is not surprising that challenges in communication and information sharing between agencies and professionals have been consistently identified in inquiries and reviews into the death or serious injury of children in the context of abuse and neglect (see DH, 1991; Reder et al, 1993; Brandon et al, 1999; Sinclair and Bullock, 2002, for systematic overviews). More recent inquiries into the deaths of children identified continuing deficits in communication and information sharing (Hammond, 2001; Laming, 2003; O'Brien, 2003). In an audit and review of Scottish child protection arrangements agencies identified the need for better communication and sharing of information (Daniel,

2004). Joint inspections of safeguarding arrangements for children in England have illustrated that agencies (and professionals) are not fully clear regarding the information that can be shared, or can be 'reluctant' to do so (DH, 2002; CSCI, 2005).

A central challenge can be the issue of confidentiality and its interpretation. Respecting confidentiality is regarded as one of the basic values and requirements for an ethical approach in social work and other professions. It appears in various professional codes of practice and ethics (BASW, 2002; Scottish Social Services Council, 2005; GMC, 2006) and the ethical complexities are discussed in various texts (for example, Clark, 2000). Professionals also are required to operate within the legal regime regulating the management of personal information (see Edwards and Rodrigues, Chapter Five, this volume). The relationship between law and ethics in the context of professional accountability in social work has been described as a 'delicate balance' (Braye and Preston-Shoot, 2006).

This chapter draws on a range of policy and legal developments and research to discuss issues of communication and information sharing in child welfare and protection. The research includes a survey undertaken by the author and colleagues of the majority of Scottish local authorities (N=29, 90% response rate) and interviews with a total of 25 social work informants drawn from three local authorities. The study explored risk assessment and interagency collaboration in the use of child protection orders by Scottish local authorities (Francis et al, 2006).[1] Child protection orders allow, among other things, for a child to be removed to or retained in a place of safety if there is the presence or risk of significant harm.

Changing policy and practice, bringing a greater emphasis on integration in the delivery of children's services, is outlined with reference to Scotland and England. Mandatory reporting laws are examined and the role of technical systems to promote information sharing and their potential to extend the surveillance and monitoring of children and families are considered.

Child protection

The 1995 Children (Scotland) Act and the 1989 Children Act in England and Wales provide the legal framework for a range of orders to investigate and intervene in family life where there is risk of significant harm to a child. Both Acts also provide the basis for service provision to children in need and focus on the one hand on supporting parents to raise their children informed by the principle of minimum intervention, while also providing for a range of compulsory measures of intervention to safeguard the welfare of children. The two Acts are underpinned by the 1998 Human Rights Act and especially Article 8 of the European Convention on Human Rights (the right to respect for private and family life).

The two Acts suggest competing philosophies in relation to the role of the state in family life and differing perspectives underlying childcare legislation have been identified (Fox Harding, 1997). The boundaries of state intervention in family life remain contested and political and public expectations are complex, with social workers expected to find the right balance between protecting children and preserving parental autonomy (Parton, 1997; Parton and Mathews, 2001). Butler and Drakeford (2005, p 80) cite an 'ebb and flow of several competing discourses around such matters as the boundary between the state and the family, the essential nature of the child ...'.

Drawing on evidence from a range of studies, Parton and Mathews (2001) indicate that in many countries child protection referrals have substantially increased. Francis et al (2006) found a 50% increase in the number of child protection orders between 1999 and 2005 (370 orders notified to the Scottish Children's Reporter Administration in 1999; 558 in 2004-05). Substance misuse, especially drug misuse (linked to pre-birth assessment), appeared to be a factor in this increase, and was identified by a number of local authorities. This rise in orders reverses a previous downward trend in the use of emergency protection measures observed in an earlier study (McGhee and Francis, 2003). Recent Scottish statistics (Scottish Executive, 2006a) note that there is a rise in neglect cases in one of the major city authorities (Glasgow) due to 'parental addiction'. Axford and Bullock (2005, p 3) observe that 'the majority of children at risk of harm present relatively low levels of abuse and neglect and are protected while living at home by means of family support services', and that the death of a child is 'relatively rare'.

The centrality of differing agencies and professionals 'working together' in ensuring effective child protection is longstanding. Daniel et al (2007), in a 'process review' of the Scottish child protection reform programme, found substantial development towards integrated approaches and 'overwhelming evidence that the principle of joint working was accepted' for child welfare and protection (p 86). Issues of accountability and agency roles and responsibilities 'for the provision of protective services' were an area where professionals identified a need for further clarity (p 87). Francis et al (2006) also found widespread acceptance of the principle of joint working among local authority social workers, although some variation in the character and nature of the arrangements for interagency and interprofessional joint working was identified. A 'lack of corporate ownership and shared responsibility for child protection practice' (Francis et al, 2006, p 9) was identified by some as a challenge to joint working. Boundary and organisational structures were sometimes seen to create additional complications in some local authorities.

Frost et al (2005), in a study of the experience of social workers in a range of multiagency children's service teams, found that boundary issues remained in place but arose at different points. White and Featherstone (2005) similarly observe that in an integrated service for child health comprising (mainly health) and social services, 'co-location did not straightforwardly lead to better communication' (p 215). Garrett (2004), in a study of the relationship between police and social workers in the specific context of child protection, observes that there is 'often a failure to interrogate what rhetorical assumptions about multi-disciplinary working actually amount to in terms of the micro-politics of "joined-up" endeavours' (p 89).

It is against this background that the question of how social workers and other professionals negotiate the sharing of information in ways that respect confidentiality for parents/carers (and children), and at the same time protect the welfare of the child, must be asked. Some of the studies below have been selected to gather information on the views of frontline social workers and other professionals. This is important as Garrett (2004) points out that the views of staff at this level are infrequently found in the 'official discourses on child welfare' (p 92).

Children's services – developments in Scotland and England

In the UK there has been renewed policy emphasis on the importance of interagency and interprofessional practice, especially in the communication and sharing of information, following the deficiencies identified in the report by Lord Laming (2003) into the death of Victoria Climbié. In Scotland a major audit and review of the child protection system (Scottish Executive, 2002) was commissioned following the fatal injury of three-year-old Kennedy McFarlane, where interagency failures in communication were identified (Hammond, 2001). Underpinning policy and organisational developments in Scotland and in England and Wales is the aim to ensure universal services address the welfare of all children and that the protection of children is a seen as a shared responsibility. The importance of sharing information for the protection and safeguarding of children's welfare is also seen as central.

In 2003 the Scottish Executive established a wide-ranging programme of reform in child protection. Several strands of development have been taken forward including guidance to build on and reinforce the role of child protection committees (Scottish Executive, 2005a) and a 'Framework of Standards' developed to support agencies in ensuring effective measures to safeguard children are in place (Scottish Executive, 2004). These are part of broader strategic developments to coordinate policy and integration in delivering children's services. Following a review of the children's hearings system, which highlighted wider issues in the delivery of children's services, planned changes at practice, organisational and legislative levels are being taken forward by the Scottish Executive as part of the *Getting it Right for Every Child* programme (Scottish Executive, 2006b). These include the development of an integrated assessment and information sharing framework to allow for multiagency assessment to ensure that children's needs are met. There has been consultation on a Children and Integrated Services Bill (Scottish Executive, 2006b). The Bill sets a legislative framework for agencies to collaborate with a broader focus on the 'well-being' of children, which includes health, welfare and development as well as considerations of harm, abuse and ill-treatment as part of the legal definition.

In England and Wales major policy, legal and organisational change is being implemented. It was first outlined in the Green Paper *Every Child Matters* (Chief Secretary to the Treasury, 2003) and is backed by new legislation (2004 Children Act). A central aim is to improve the coordination and integration of services to children and families and to safeguard children within the context of universal services, essentially to 'mainstream child protection within a universal children's services framework' (O'Brien et al, 2006, p 379). The focus is on the 'well-being' of children, ensuring that all children have access to universal services and that additional needs are addressed alongside effective measures to protect children. The importance of early intervention to prevent later difficulties arising is emphasised. Children's trusts are being established to ensure a greater integration of services, and local safeguarding boards replace area child protection committees to ensure effective measures to protect children at risk of harm. A central element of the reforms is to ensure that information sharing and assessment is significantly improved. There are new duties on agencies to cooperate and all agencies are required to take account of the need to safeguard children in carrying out their functions.

It is these developing arrangements that will set the structure for interagency and interprofessional collaboration in meeting the needs of children, including any need for protection.

Information sharing – confidentiality, communication and trust

Children's services

Extensive government guidance, interagency protocols and professional ethical and statutory codes on sharing information provide guidance where a child may be at risk of harm (Scottish Office, 1998; Scottish Executive, 2003; DfES, 2006a; GMC, 2006). However, uncertainties can arise about what information to share and when to share it. These are related to issues of interpretation and assessment as well as levels of certainty. Lupton et al (2001), for example, found more 'conflict and doubt' in general practitioners (GPs) when 'vague suspicions' rather than firm convictions were in place. As Munro (2005, p 380) indicates, inquiries have consistently shown that 'much of the relevant information in child protection is ambiguous, open to interpretation as sinister or benign'. Scottish good practice guidance recognises some of the complexities, stating that '[d]ecisions about when to involve other agencies, when to breach confidentiality and when to refer to the children's reporter, are difficult and complex' (Scottish Executive, 2003, p 1).

Professional understandings regarding the nature and extent of confidentiality are relevant. Sinclair and Bullock (2002), in an analysis of 40 serious case reviews (formal reviews instigated where a child died or suffered serious injury where abuse or neglect was a significant feature), found inadequate sharing of information as practitioners were unclear about confidentiality and consent; concerns about breaching data protection law were also present. The Laming Report (2003) found that unless concerns were clearly labelled as 'child protection', fear of breaching data protection and human rights law inhibited the sharing of information and thus limited effective assessment. Francis et al (2006) found social work interviewees articulated some 'frustration' in relation to a lack of consistent practice in sharing information and variability between agencies; different understandings and views about confidentiality remained a factor. Differing professional views on 'responsibilities to adults in child protection cases' (p 10) and in balancing the rights of the child and the parent(s) were germane. Daniel et al (2007) found a more positive picture with a few social workers surveyed expressing concern about other agencies but many more indicating improved information sharing and increased referral raising resource issues.

O'Brien et al (2006) have reported recent findings from the first stage of a national evaluation of children's trusts (part of the new arrangements for agencies to collaborate in England in providing children's services). They found information sharing protocols were less well developed, compared with other strategic dimensions such as arrangements to cooperate on governance, with only 15 out of 35 'pathfinders' having information sharing protocols in place. They indicate that 'concerns remained about sharing confidential information across professional groupings' (p 389) despite the importance of this dimension for integrated service provision.

Health and adult services

There are complexities in the interface between adult and child services in the context of safeguarding children. This may be partly related to more limited knowledge and understanding regarding children's needs on the part of some adult service practitioners. As one respondent in a Scottish local authority survey concisely observed, 'practitioners in adult services were less skilled at recognising when their client's difficulties can have a negative effect on the care of their children' (Francis et al, 2006, p 22). The report of the inquiry into the death of 11-week-old Caleb Ness (O'Brien, 2003) identified specific issues in the border between child and adult services. There was also a failure of criminal justice services (which are primarily located in local authorities, there being no separate probation service in Scotland) to recognise their child protection responsibilities. Daniel et al (2007), in their review of the Scottish child protection reform programme, found that criminal justice and community care social workers embarking on child protection training 'expressed concern and anxiety about their role and responsibilities' in this area (p 15), although key informants perceived positive improvement in the interface between adult and criminal justice services.

These complexities are probably most exemplified in health-related settings. Sharing information to assess risk at the time of child protection order applications is important and several Scottish local authorities surveyed (Francis et al, 2006) identified no major difficulties in gathering the required information, with health visitors, alongside police, most commonly providing information (93%, N=27). Lupton et al (1999), in a study of the National Health Service (NHS) and child protection networks, found that health visitors were seen as having a key role in child protection by 81% of frontline staff in the NHS. Some ongoing challenges in gathering information from health professionals and GPs were identified by several Scottish local authorities most likely related to concerns about breach of confidentiality (Francis et al, 2006). The role of GPs has remained a consistent issue in child protection and in relation to children in need (Stevenson, 1999). Lupton et al (1999) found that GPs were clear about their role in child protection although some saw this as more limited compared with other professional groups and most relevant at identification and pre-referral stages.

Parental drug abuse has been estimated as affecting between 40,000 and 60,000 children in Scotland (University of Glasgow, 2002). Drug advice services were reported as a source of information in child protection order applications by some Scottish local authorities (24%, N=27; Francis et al, 2006). Taylor and Kroll (2004), as part of a wider study of child welfare and parental substance misuse, explored some of the tensions and dilemmas facing practitioners in adult and children's services where parental drug and alcohol misuse is present. For many childcare workers interviewed (social work and family centre staff), specialist drug workers were seen to focus on the adult client and issues of maintaining trust and confidentiality could at times overcome the principle of the paramountcy of the child's welfare. Moreover, a number of 'childcare social workers' thought that there was a lack of understanding of the importance of gaining information and of breaching confidentiality in 'high-risk cases' where this was necessary in the interests of the child (p 1122).

Kearney et al (2003), in a major review of the interface between services where there are parental mental health, drug or alcohol difficulties, found similar differences in understandings about confidentiality between social services and medical colleagues, especially consultant psychiatrists. Richardson and Asthana (2006), drawing on a range of studies on information sharing generally in health and social care, observed that 'profound differences in professional culture exist' (p 662), although they pointed out that there is limited information on 'the role of professional culture in inter-agency information sharing' (p 665). Lupton et al (2001) observed tensions around sharing information and issues of power and status in child protection. There was recognition from some interviewees in a Scottish study that there had been some change in the health sector with a greater willingness to share information than in the past (Francis et al, 2006).

Thresholds and perspectives

Axford and Bullock (2005, p 8) emphasise that an underpinning requirement for an effective child protection service is a 'common language' between professionals involved with children that provides for shared meaning and agreed terms. In Francis et al's (2006) study, several Scottish local authorities identified a 'lack of shared perspectives on child protection' (p 22) as a contributory factor to less effective interagency practice in child protection. This partly related to issues of thresholds for intervention and clearly this is an area where differing interprofessional perspectives can arise. A report into the abuse and neglect of children in a family with extensive service involvement reported that health and social services had differing views on the level of risk to the child (SWIA, 2005, p 9). Munro (2005) cited evidence that professionals do disagree significantly in assessing what constitutes abuse. Daniel (2004) noted in a Scottish audit and review of child protection practice that education and health staff frequently considered that social work did not take their referrals sufficiently seriously. Lupton et al (1999) similarly found that some health professionals considered social services as 'slow' in responding. This was related to apparent differing thresholds for intervention. Frost et al (2005) observe that, in general, agencies set their own criteria for referrals to gatekeep boundaries to manage resources and focus on 'core aims'.

Communication

Information sharing is not synonymous with effective communication or accurate assessment of risk. The report *An Inspection into the Care and Protection of Children in Eilean Siar* (SWIA, 2005) observed that agencies within Eilean Siar (Western Isles) 'shared information constantly about the family, both in and outwith formal meetings' (p 10) but implications were not fully assessed or discussed by the professionals involved. In an analysis of 45 inquiry reports between 1973 and 1994, all but two examining the death or serious injury of children in the context of abuse and neglect, Munro (1998) differentiated between poor assessment and 'failure to collect information' (p 90). She observed in later inquiries substantially fewer critiques of social workers in the latter area, although concerns about assessment remained.

Munro (2005) contends that in child protection practice major difficulties lie in the 'psychological complexities of communicating effectively' (p 383). Reder and Duncan (2003) argue for the importance of understanding the 'psychology of communication' and that in child abuse inquiries the major psychological issues were not practical but 'how professionals thought about the case, processed the information available to them and interacted with other informants' (p 83). They argue that professionals need to develop core skills in communication – what they refer to as a 'communication mindset' – and that the ethos 'I am part of a system' needs to become an automatic approach to thinking about their work in this context.

Brandon et al (1999), in an analysis of serious child abuse cases in Wales, found that a significant element in communication failures was a lack of respect or mistrust of the perspectives of other professionals. Francis et al (2006) similarly found that trust and confidence were important to joint working and information sharing at both interagency and interprofessional levels in child protection work. While policy and procedures were seen to support the development of confidence, the quality of individual working relationships was considered important to effective information sharing and collaboration. Police and health visitors are key partners within the UK child protection process and relationships tend to be viewed positively (Lupton et al 1999; Francis et al, 2006), most likely reflecting their central role in investigation. O'Brien et al (2006) found in their children's trusts pathfinders study that the development of trust and knowledge of other professional expertise was central to good information sharing.

Hudson (2005) points to the importance of culture and differences in power and status in the context of arrangements to share information generally in multidisciplinary teams and argues that for this to be effective a 'climate of interprofessional trust and mutual respect' is required (p 545). Brown and White (2006), reviewing general evidence regarding the integration of children's services, highlight some potential barriers, including differences in professional culture, role clarity and professional boundaries.

These findings serve to illustrate some of the complexities underpinning issues of communication and information sharing in child protection policy and practice, including issues around differing professionals' perspectives on confidentiality.

Mandatory reporting

Several jurisdictions have mandatory reporting laws requiring professionals to inform child protection services of suspected abuse. These include the US, Canada, Australia (apart from Western Australia) and Denmark (Kalichman, 1999; Harries and Clare, 2002; Ainsworth and Hansen, 2006). Mandatory reporting legislation is often seen as a solution to failures to share information by overriding the legal and ethical reasons for non-reporting of suspected or actual abuse by a range of professionals.

In the US, mandatory reporting laws emerged in the mid-1960s, coinciding with the identification of the 'battered child syndrome' (Kempe et al, 1962) and awareness that physicians were reluctant to report abuse by parents (Kalichman, 1999). Mandatory reporting laws have given rise to much debate and controversy. Harries and Clare (2002), summarising evidence in this area, observe that 'many of the arguments are polemical and most of the "evidence" inferential and presumptive' (p 31).

Kalichman (1999) provides a detailed analysis of legal and ethical issues in the US, summarising debates surrounding these provisions. Definitional problems within statutes arise in terms of both legal definitions of abuse and required levels of belief or suspicion (Myers, 1992, cited in Flaherty, 2006; Kalichman, 1999). Levine (1998, cited in Kalichman, 1999) found that child protection workers had a more restricted definition of 'reasonable cause to suspect abuse' compared with mental health professionals. In a national audit of child protection research in Australia, Higgins et al (2005) found that there was a need to provide 'education and support' especially to health and education professionals 'to better understand when they needed to make a report' (p 33). It is clear that professionals' ethical concerns, issues of risk, weighing in some cases a perceived potential greater harm of reporting, and lack of service response by child protection agencies all intertwine in the decision to report or in some cases not to report (Kalichman, 1999).

Mandatory reporting is associated with increases in notification (Harries and Clare, 2002) and the incidence of non-substantiated reports (Besharov, 1990, cited in Bell and Tooman, 1994; Ainsworth, 2002; Ainsworth and Hansen, 2006). Kalichman (1999) indicates that this is a common critique expressed by opponents of mandatory reporting; overreporting of suspected abuse and the costs of investigation can impact on direct resources for prevention and intervention where abuse and neglect are present. Benefits of mandatory reporting are seen as including increased reporting; clear responsibility on all professionals to report suspected abuse; and a greater understanding of child protection (Bell and Tooman, 1994). However, Harries and Clare (2002, p 49) contend that 'There is no evidence that mandatory reporting increases the quality, quantity or benefits to children who are 'at risk of harm' or to families who are vulnerable. Indeed there is some evidence that it does the reverse'.

In Scotland there is a duty on local authorities to investigate and bring to the attention of the reporter to the children's hearing any child where there appears to be a need for compulsory measures of supervision (1995 Children (Scotland) Act 1995, section 53). There is, of course, formal guidance and interagency child protection procedures to ensure that child abuse concerns are reported to the relevant agencies. The Scottish Executive plans to issue a non-statutory Code of Practice on sharing information to protect children with the intention of underpinning this with statutory duties (Harvie-Clark, 2007). In England and Wales new provisions for children's databases have caused much controversy (see below).

Children's databases

The influence of information and communication technology (ICT) on social work is part of wider debates about the development of the 'surveillance society' and the impact at both individual and societal levels of 'large-scale technological infrastructures' (Ball and Wood, 2006, p 1). Gallagher (2005), in the editorial of a special technology-focused issue of *Child Abuse Review*, poses the general question as to whether 'new technology is helping or harming children' (p 367), and how to reduce any harm and take advantage of the positives in the application of new technology. Garrett (2005, p 541) argues that 'a greater reliance on databases and other e-technologies risks promoting the idea that complex problems relating to children and families requiring child welfare services can be quickly solved'. Evans and Harris (2004, p 70), moreover, argue that the emphasis on risk is 'shifting the parameters of the debate about confidentiality from a question of citizenship rights to an aspect of social order'.

In England, section 12 of the 2004 Children Act provides for the setting up of children's databases. Much of the recent debate around the use of ICT has focused on such databases, especially the planned Information Sharing Index (now called ContactPoint) authorised by the Act, and the potential for the extension of social surveillance to wider populations of children and families (Garrett, 2005; Munro, 2005; Penna, 2005; Anderson et al, 2006). The Index will ultimately provide a record of all children in England. It is expected to contain basic identification information (name, address, gender, date of birth, parent(s)/carer(s), GP, school) and the contact details of any professionals providing 'specialist or targeted services' (apart from 'sensitive services', which include sexual health, mental health and substance abuse services where consent is required unless the child is suffering or at risk of suffering 'significant harm'), and it was envisaged that practitioners could indicate that they have 'important information to share', or 'have undertaken an assessment under the common assessment framework' or 'taken any action relating to the person' (Draft Information Sharing Index (England) Regulations 2007, regs 4, 5 and Schedule 1). The Index is described as 'an important tool to help improve the communication between key professionals needed for the effective delivery of services for children and families and, when necessary, to protect children' (DfES, 2006b, para 2). Extensive guidance on the 2004 Act is in place, including sharing information (HM Government, 2006a, 2006b) and interagency working to protect children (DfES, 2006a).

Munro and Parton (2007) have contended that the register in effect is a form of mandatory reporting with a broader criterion than suspicion or belief of child abuse, and that this may have some of the deleterious impact that has been identified with mandatory reporting. This includes the potential for increased reporting of information but not necessarily a commensurate increase in services; moreover, cooperation and willingness to seek help can be adversely affected by limited confidentiality. The Index will provide information on basic contact details and the current principles of sharing information will apply when practitioners make contact with another agency. However, Munro and Parton (2007, p 13) argue that a further 'somewhat vague additional criterion' to share information is in place in government guidance in addition to the traditional presence or risk of significant harm. The final regulations[2] have removed the need for subjective judgements by practitioners as to whether they have 'important information' or action to report. This now may address some of the concerns outlined by Munro and Parton (2007). There is clearly the opportunity for better coordination of services but the potential for 'function creep' and increased intervention and regulation by the state in family life also exist.

Conclusion

Protecting children requires effective communication between professionals and agencies. This is important in coming to an assessment of risk, as the collation of information and observations provides a clearer picture of any significant patterns in the child's circumstances. This is accepted in UK child protection practice and challenges to effective communication are recognised. Some of the continuing challenges and complexities that impact on effective communication and information sharing have been outlined in this chapter and revolve around interprofessional and interagency collaboration, professional differences and understandings of confidentiality, issues of common standards or frameworks to make sense of information and differing thresholds for intervention between professionals. The importance of trust between professionals for effective communication and collaboration is emphasised in building collaborative networks.

Mandatory reporting laws do not provide a straightforward solution to the ethical and legal barriers often cited as inhibiting the sharing of confidential information. They can create over-reporting as substantial numbers of referrals are found to be unsubstantiated, with potential consequent impact on resources available for prevention and intervention. Moreover, the efficacy of these types of legal frameworks in improving outcomes for children and families appears to be unproven.

The implications of ICT have yet to be fully explored in professional practice with children and families. The creation of a major database containing information on all children in England (at present) may allow for better coordination of services but this has to be balanced against the potential costs to the privacy rights of children and their families. As with mandatory reporting legislation the question will be whether the database supports beneficial outcomes for children and their families, leading to better access to services and support when needed or potentially serves to extend greater surveillance and monitoring to ever larger numbers of children.

Besides effective communication and sharing of information, protecting children ultimately requires well-trained and skilled practitioners who can synthesise this information and who have sufficient time and access to resources to undertake direct work to support children and their families. Developments in England and Scotland aim to provide better integration in the delivery of children's services including protective services. The ultimate test, however, of any child welfare system remains whether it serves to provide for better outcomes for children.

Notes

[1] The study was sponsored by the Scottish Executive and the views expressed in the (research) report (Francis et al, 2006) are those of the authors and do not necessarily reflect the views of the Scottish Executive or any other organisation(s) by which the authors are employed. The views expressed in this chapter are those of the author.

[2] The 2007 Children Act Information 2004 Database (England) Regulations, SI 2007/2182.

References

Ainsworth, F. (2002) 'Mandatory reporting of child abuse and neglect: does it really make a difference?', *Child and Family Social Work*, vol 7, pp 57–63.

Ainsworth, F. and Hansen, P. (2006) 'Five tumultuous years in Australian child protection: little progress', *Child and Family Social Work*, vol 11, pp 33–41.

Anderson, R., Brown, I., Clayton, R., Dowty, T., Korff, D. and Munro, E. (2006) *Children's Databases – Safety and Privacy. A Report for the Information Commissioner*, Foundation for Information Policy Research, www.ico.gov.uk/upload/documents/library/data_protection/detailed_specialist_guides/ico_issues_paper_protecting_chidrens_personal_information.pdf

Axford, N. and Bullock, R. (2005) *Child Death and Significant Case Review: International Approaches*, Dartington Social Research Unit, Insight 19, Edinburgh: Scottish Executive Education Department.

Ball, K. and Wood, D.M. (eds) (2006) *A Report on the Surveillance Society for the Information Commissioner by the Surveillance Society Network: Summary Report*, www.ico.gov.uk/upload/documents/library/data_protection/practical_application/surveillance_society_summary_06.pdf

BASW (British Association of Social Workers) (2002) *The Code of Ethics for Social Work*, Birmingham: BASW.

Bell, L. and Tooman, P. (1994) 'Mandatory reporting laws: a critical overview', *International Journal of Law and the Family*, vol, 8, pp 337–56.

Besharov, D. (1990) *Recognizing Child Abuse: A Guide for the Concerned*, New York: The Free Press, cited in Bell, L. and Tooman, P. (1994) 'Mandatory reporting laws: a critical overview', *International Journal of Law and the Family*, vol, 8, pp 337–56.

Brandon, M., Owers, M. and Black, J. (1999) *Learning How to Make Children Safer: An Analysis for the Welsh Office of Serious Child Abuse Cases in Wales*, Norwich: Centre for Research on the Child and Family, University of East Anglia.

Braye, S. and Preston-Shoot, M. (2006) 'The role of law in welfare reform: critical perspectives on the relationship between law and social work practice', *International Journal of Social Welfare*, vol 15, pp 19–26.

Brown, K. and White, K. (2006) *Exploring the Evidence Base for Integrated Children's Services*, Edinburgh: Scottish Executive Education Department, www.scotland.gov.uk/Resource/Doc/90282/0021746.pdf

Butler, I. and Drakeford, M. (2005) *Scandal, Social Policy and Social Welfare* (2nd edition), Bristol: The Policy Press.

Chief Secretary to the Treasury (2003) *Every Child Matters*, Cm 5860, London: The Stationery Office.

Clark, C.L. (2000) *Social Work Ethics: Politics, Principles and Practice*, Basingstoke: Palgrave.

Crichton, J.H.M. (2001) 'Confidentiality: guidance from the General Medical Council and the Royal College of Psychiatrists', *The Journal of Forensic Psychiatry*, vol 12, no 3, pp 671-6.

CSCI (Commission for Social Care Inspection) (2005) *Safeguarding Children: The Second Joint Chief Inspector's Report on Arrangements to Safeguard Children*, Newcastle: CSCI.

Daniel, B. (2004) 'An overview of the Scottish multidisciplinary child protection review', *Child and Family Social Work*, vol 9, pp 247-57.

Daniel, B., Vincent, S. and Ogilvie-Whyte, S. (2007) *A Process Review of the Child Protection Reform Programme*, Edinburgh: Scottish Executive Social Research.

DfES (Department for Education and Skills) (2006a) *Working Together to Safeguard Children: A Guide to Inter-Agency Working to Safeguard and Promote the Welfare of Children*, London: DfES.

DfES (2006b) *Information Sharing Index: Consultation on Draft Information Sharing Index (England) Regulations and Partial Regulatory Impact Assessment*, www.everychildmatters.gov.uk/delivering services/contactpoint/legislation/

DH (Department of Health) (1991) *Child Abuse: A Study of Inquiry Reports 1980-1989*, London: HMSO.

DH (1995) *Child Protection Messages from Research*, London: HMSO.

DH (2002) *Safeguarding Children: A Joint Chief Inspectors' Report on Arrangements to Safeguard Children*, London: DH.

DHSS (Department of Health and Social Services) (1974) *Report of the Committee of Inquiry into the Care and Supervision Provided in Relation to Maria Colwell*, London: HMSO.

Evans, T. and Harris, J. (2004) 'Citizenship, social inclusion and confidentiality', *British Journal of Social Work*, vol 34, pp 69-91.

Flaherty, E. (2006) 'Does the wording of the mandate to report suspected child abuse serve as another barrier to child abuse reporting?', *Child Abuse and Neglect*, vol 30, pp 341-3.

Fox Harding, L. (1997) *Perspectives in Child Care Policy* (2nd edition), Harlow: Addison Wesley Longman Limited.

Francis, J., McGhee, J. and Mordaunt, E. (2006) *Protecting Children in Scotland: An Investigation of Risk Assessment and Inter-agency Collaboration in the Use of Child Protection Orders*, Edinburgh: Scottish Executive Social Research, web-only report, www.scotland.gov. uk/Publications/2006/05/SprPrCis

Frost, N., Robinson, M. and Anning, A. (2005) 'Social workers in multidisciplinary teams: issues and dilemmas for professional practice', *Child and Family Social Work*, vol 10, pp 187-96.

Gallagher, B. (2005) 'New technology: helping or harming children?', Editorial, *Child Abuse Review*, vol 14, pp 367-73.

Garrett, P.M. (2004) 'Talking child protection: the police and social workers "working together"', *Journal of Social Work*, vol 4, no 1, pp 77-97.

Garrett, P.M. (2005) 'Social work's "electronic turn": notes on the deployment of information and communication technologies in social work with children and families', *Critical Social Policy*, vol 25, no 4, pp 529-53.

GMC (General Medical Council) (2006) *Good Medical Practice*, www. gmc-uk.org/guidance/good_medical_practice/index/asp

Hallett, C. and Birchall, E. (1992) *Coordination and Child Protection: A Review of the Literature*, Edinburgh: HMSO.

Hammond, H. (2001) *Child Protection Inquiry into the Circumstances Surrounding the Death of Kennedy McFarlane, d.o.b. 17 April 1997*, Dumfries and Galloway Child Protection Committee, www.dumgal. gov.uk/services/depts/SocialServices/acrobat/CPEnquiry.pdf

Harries, M. and Clare, M. (2002) *Mandatory Reporting of Child Abuse: Evidence and Opinions, Report Prepared by the University of Western Australia, Discipline of Social Work and Social Policy*, July, Perth: Western Australia Child Protection Council.

Harvie-Clark, S. (2007) *Protection of Vulnerable Groups (Scotland) Bill: Parliamentary Consideration Prior to Stage 3*, Edinburgh: Scottish Parliament Information Centre (SPICe).

Higgins, D.J., Adams, R.M., Bromfield, L., Richardson, N. and Aldana, M. (2005) *National Audit of Australian Child Protection Research 1995-2004*, National Child Protection Clearinghouse, Australian Institute of Family Studies, Commissioned by Australian Centre for Child Protection, University of South Australia, www.unisa.edu. au/childprotection/publications.asp

HM Government (2006a) *Information Sharing: Practitioners' Guide, Integrated Working to Improve Outcomes for Children and Young People*, London: DfES, www.everychildmatters.gov.uk/resources-and-practice/IG00065.

HM Government (2006b) *Information Sharing: Further Guidance on Legal Issues*, London: DfES, www.everychildmatters.gov.uk/resources-and-practice/IG00065/

Hudson, B. (2005) 'Information sharing and children's services reform in England: can legislation change practice?', *Journal of Interprofessional Care*, vol 19, no 6, pp 537-46.

Kalichman, S. (1999) *Mandatory Reporting of Suspected Child Abuse, Ethics, Law and Policy* (2nd edition), Washington, DC: American Psychological Association.

Kearney, P., Levin, E. and Rosen, G. (2003) *Alcohol, Drug and Mental Health Problems: Working with Families*, Report No. 2, London: Social Care Institute for Excellence.

Kempe, C., Silverman, S., Steele, B., Doegmuller, W. and Silver, H. (1962) 'The battered child syndrome', *Journal of the American Medical Association*, vol 181, pp 4-11.

Laming, Lord (2003) *The Victoria Climbié Inquiry*, Cm 5730, London: The Stationery Office..

Levine, M. (1998) 'Do standards of proof affect decision making in child protection investigations?', *Law and Human Behaviour*, vol 22, pp 341-7, cited in Kalichman, S. (1999) *Mandatory Reporting of Suspected Child Abuse, Ethics, Law and Policy* (2nd edition), Washington, DC: American Psychological Association.

Lupton, C., North, N. and Khan, P. (2001) *Working Together or Pulling Apart? The National Health Service and Child Protection Network*, Bristol: The Policy Press.

Lupton, C., Khan, P., North, N. and Lacey, D. (1999) *The Role of Health Professionals in the Child Protection Process*, Portsmouth: Portsmouth Social Services Research and Information Unit, University of Portsmouth.

McGhee, J. and Francis, J. (2003) 'Protecting children in Scotland: examining the impact of the Children (Scotland) Act 1995', *Child and Family Social Work*, vol 8, pp 133-42.

Munro, E. (1998) 'Improving social workers' knowledge base in child protection work', *British Journal of Social Work*, vol 28, pp 89-105.

Munro, E. (2005) 'What tools do we need to improve identification of child abuse', *Child Abuse Review*, vol 14, pp 374-88.

Munro, E. and Parton, N. (2007) 'How far is England in the process of introducing a mandatory reporting system?', *Child Abuse Review*, vol 16, pp 5-16.

Myers, J.E.B. (1992) *Legal Issues in Child Abuse and Neglect*, Newbury Park, CA: Sage Publications, cited in Flaherty, E. (2006) 'Does the wording of the mandate to report suspected child abuse serve as another barrier to child abuse reporting?', *Child Abuse and Neglect*, vol 30, pp 341-3.

O'Brien, M., Bachmann, M., Husbands, C., Shreeve, A., Jones, N., Watson, J. and Shemilt, I. (2006) 'Integrating children's services to promote children's welfare: early findings from the implementation of the Children's Trusts in England', *Child Abuse Review*, vol 15, pp 377-95.

O'Brien, S. (2003) *Report of the Caleb Ness Inquiry*, Edinburgh: Edinburgh and the Lothians Child Protection Committee.

Parton, N. (ed) (1997) *Child Protection and Family Support: Tensions, Contradictions and Possibilities*, London: Routledge.

Parton, N. and Mathews, R. (2001) 'New direction in child protection and family support in Western Australia: a policy initiative to re-focus child welfare practice', *Child and Family Social Work*, vol 6, pp 97-113.

Penna, S. (2005) 'The Children Act 2004: child protection and social surveillance', *Journal of Social Welfare and Family Law*, vol 27, no 2, pp 43-157.

Reder, P. and Duncan, S. (2003) 'Understanding communication in child protection networks', *Child Abuse Review*, vol 12, pp 82-100.

Reder, P., Duncan, S. and Gray, M. (1993) *Beyond Blame: Child Abuse Tragedies Revisited*, London: Routledge.

Richardson, S. and Asthana, S. (2006) 'Inter-agency information and sharing in health and social care services: The role of professinal culture', *British Journal of Social Work*, vol 36, pp 657-69.

Scottish Executive (2002) *'It's Everyone's Job to Make Sure I'm Alright': Report of the Child Protection Audit and Review*, Edinburgh: Scottish Executive.

Scottish Executive (2003) *Sharing Information about Children at Risk: A Guide to Good Practice*, Edinburgh: Scottish Executive.

Scottish Executive (2004) *Protecting Children and Young People: Framework for Standards*, Edinburgh: Scottish Executive.

Scottish Executive (2005a) *Protecting Children and Young People: Child Protection Committees*, Edinburgh: Scottish Executive.

Scottish Executive (2005b) *Children's Social Work Statistics*, Edinburgh: Scottish Executive, www.scotland.gov.uk/ Publications/2005/10/2791127/11278

Scottish Executive (2006a) *Child Protection Statistics 2005-06*, National Statistics Publication, Health and Social Care Series, Edinburgh: Scottish Executive, www.scotland.gov.uk/Resource/ Doc/149835/0039892.pdf

Scottish Executive (2006b) *Getting it Right for Every Child*, Draft Children's Services (Scotland) Bill Consultation, Edinburgh: Scottish Executive.

Scottish Office (1998) *Protecting Children: A Shared Responsibility. Guidance on Inter-Agency Co-operation*, Edinburgh: Scottish Office.

Scottish Social Services Council (2005) *Code of Practice for Social Service Workers*, Dundee: Scottish Social Services Council.

Sinclair, R. and Bullock, R. (2002) *Learning from Past Experience: A Review of Serious Case Reviews*, London: Department of Health.

Stevenson, O. (1999) 'Children in need and abused: interprofessional and interagency responses', in O. Stevenson (ed) *Child Welfare in the United Kingdom 1948-1998*, Oxford: Blackwell Science, pp 100-20.

SWIA (Social Work Inspection Agency) (2005) *An Inspection into the Care and Protection of Children in Eilean Siar*, Edinburgh: Scottish Executive.

Taylor, A. and Kroll, B. (2004) 'Working with parental substance misuse: dilemmas for practice', *British Journal of Social Work*, vol 34, no 8, pp 1115-32.

University of Glasgow Centre for Drug Misuse Research (2002) *Parental Drug Misuse in Scotland*, Glasgow: University of Glasgow.

Waterhouse, L. and McGhee, J. (2002) 'Social work with children and families', in R. Adams, L. Dominelli and M. Payne (eds) *Social Work: Themes, Issues and Critical Debates* (2nd edition), Basingstoke: Palgrave with the Open University, pp 267-86.

White, S. and Featherstone, B. (2005) 'Communicating misunderstandings: multi-agency work as social practice', *Child and Family Social Work*, vol 10, no 3, pp 207-16.

NINE

Working with children and young people: privacy and identity

Peter Ashe

Introduction

Some years ago, we were waiting in an airport arrivals area for our teenage son to return from the other side of the world. After a lengthy and fruitless wait alongside the baggage carousel, we decided to ask where he might be. At the domestic airline desk we were solemnly informed that 'under the terms of the [1998] Data Protection Act, such private information could not be released'. Other than suggest that we *could* ask the police to force him to tell us, the official seemed unable to do anything other than repeat this simple mantra. Luckily, the call-handler at the international airline involved in the journey had been trained to deal with such transactions within the frame of customer relations first, and the Data Protection Act second. We were able to establish our bona fides, and with a helpful piece of smoothing, 'yes, I know, parents are often very anxious in these circumstances', she went to check for us. It transpired that our son was safe and somewhere over Honolulu at the time. We were a day early to meet him – we had got the international date-line the wrong way round.

By that time I had already spent several years working on information sharing and its governance, and this was a wonderfully salutary lesson for me in how things can spiral away from contact with reality – who could have thought that the first airline's mantra was a remotely satisfactory way to relate to anxious parents? Only someone who spent all their time at HQ worrying about corporate liability, it seemed.

At the other end of this range of practice, I had been very pleasantly surprised by some anecdotal feedback from one of the pioneer information sharing projects within the national 'eCare' programme on data sharing. Working with older people on Single Shared Assessments (SEHD, 2001), practitioners had taken care to explain what would happen with their clients' and patients' personal information, and found that the ensuing discussion had often elided into an explanation of how services worked together in the system. The practitioners acknowledged that they had previously tended not to have this sort of conversation, and they felt that although the new dialogue took some extra time, older service users had a much better understanding of what they were experiencing as a result.

There is currently much public debate about identity, information sharing between public agencies, and privacy. This chapter comprises some personal reflections on what might be thought to be the simple process of talking to people about their personal information, and how public agencies (generally in Scotland, but also elsewhere in the UK) have handled and are handling it. As I am currently working mostly on children's services, that is what this chapter is focused on, but it is informed by my experience generally.

The chapter first sketches the longstanding policy emphasis on person- or child-centred services and its recent critique. Next, some of the substantial volume of recent consultation with children and young people about the use of their personal information is briefly discussed. The chapter asks whether current approaches offer a sustainable framework for the near future. The 'privacy pragmatism' approach first propounded in the Cabinet Office report on information sharing (6, 2002) is considered as a potential theoretical prop, together with 'personal learning planning' as a potential fulcrum, for the bridge-building I see as necessary if information sharing practice is to take account of rapidly developing trends in the lived experiences of children and young people. I suggest that if we reframe our consideration of this issue we may have an opportunity to build towards a sustainable set of social relationships between people, their personal data, and its public custodians.

Privacy and children

Shareable personal information is increasingly seen as integral to the effective delivery of important public services. Information sharing throws new light on familiar discourse on liberties and rights, especially privacy. Privacy seems important to people generally, and with its protective and empowering functions, especially so to children and young people. Some see new approaches to information handling, in particular the sharing of information between agencies, as supporting a broader move to regulate and control children.

In 2006 the Foundation for Information Policy Research (FIPR) was asked by the Information Commissioner to critique the recent development of large-scale children's databases (Anderson et al, 2006). It suggested that the working out of privacy is a deeply significant enabler of children's development as autonomous social beings, in an evolving relationship with the people and institutions around them:

Privacy is the mechanism by which we define who we are in relation to other people, and as such can be seen as an essential element of child welfare and child protection because it encourages the development of clear personal boundaries. Indeed, many writers on the subject have stressed the vital nature of privacy in self-development and self-definition:

> Privacy is necessary to the creation of selves out of human beings, since a self is at least in part a human being who regards his existence, his thoughts, his body, his actions as his own. (Anderson et al, 2006, p 109)

The FIPR report (Anderson et al, 2006, p 109), quotes Westin (2003):

> Changing personal needs and choices about self-revelation are what make privacy such a complex condition, and a matter of personal choice. The importance of that right to choose, both to the individual's self-development and to the exercise of responsible citizenship, makes the claim to privacy a fundamental part of civil liberty in democratic society. If we are 'switched on' without our knowledge or consent, we have lost our rights to decide when and with whom we speak, publish, worship and associate (Westin, 2003).

Finally, the point is made that adult respect for children's privacy is an excellent promoter of child protection in its broader sense:

> Developing a sense of privacy and autonomy in relation to one's personal life is an integral part of becoming a distinct individual. It is thus important that adults maintain a scrupulous respect for privacy in their dealings with children, in order to reinforce personal boundaries and underline each child's right to say 'no' to unwanted intrusion. In this way, the right to privacy directly empowers children to protect themselves. (Anderson et al, 2006, p 109)

Policy development and its critique

The main UK-wide social policy drivers on information sharing were outlined in a major privacy project funded by the Economic and Social Research Council Society Today programme (ESRC, 2003–05), where Chris Bellamy and others joined Charles Raab and Perri 6 in building (6 et al, 2004, 2005a) on their pathfinding work for the Cabinet Office in 2002 (PIU, 2002). These drivers may be summarised as:

- the development of social intervention programmes involving a focus on extremely small neighbourhoods, groups or individuals, together with a shift towards holistic, multiagency approaches to such interventions;
- strategies for managing rationing in a number of key services as a corollary of establishing of ambitious social policies at a time of continuing resource constraint;
- the government's response to administrative discretion in a policy context calling for more finely judged selectivity; and the desire to base interventions on more precise evidence;
- an increased priority given to preventive approaches to managing risk;
- a focus on social exclusion, while placing an enhanced emphasis on the obligations of citizenship; this is a manifestation of a communitarian strand within policy, wherein antisocial behaviour, failure to parent, benefit fraud and so on are seen as being at the root of many social ills, and those involved, or at risk of being so, should be identified. (from 6 et al, 2005a, and Bellamy et al, 2005)

One can see some of these drivers echoed within the FIPR's critique of the development of children's databases, with the implications for privacy and shareable information (Anderson et al, 2006). These databases represent a shift away from the previous 'residual and reactive' stance. The FIPR sees the move towards general prevention of problems for children as borrowed from crime prevention (although the causal chain is not so clear or robust as there). Also borrowed is the idea that offending and antisocial behaviour are linked and can be prevented. The shift from universal to targeted preventive services and policy development has proceeded with general agreement that the population-based approach is acceptable. The FIPR identifies that targeted prevention is appropriate to stop things getting worse.

The other major shift that the FIPR identifies is a move from *protection* to *safeguarding*. In brief, it suggests that this involves the application of child protection principles (involving about 50,000 children at risk of significant harm) to general welfare needs (where between three and four million children are thought to be at some disadvantage) (DH, 2000). An active interventionist approach to family life in order to prevent problems developing has created a 'managerial framework for children's development, with an audit system of targets and performance indicators' (Anderson et al, 2006, p 13). Responsibility for achieving targets has been given to professionals in children's services, and this consequently leads to a fundamental reduction in the autonomy and privacy of family life. The data implications of this are summarised as

> The shift from universal to targeted services, where the need for additional help is identified by professionals rather than parents, creates the drive for extensive data collection so that agencies can build up a wide-ranging picture of a child's functioning. (Anderson et al, 2006, p 15).

Consultation with children

Alongside policy development there is a strong emphasis on consultation with children and young people. The authors of *Young Children's Citizenship* found:

> There seems to be no limit to the type of methods used, from conventional research techniques to the most creative and fun-based activities imaginable. Playworkers, teachers, social workers, civil servants, housing managers and commercial organisations are seeking the views and ideas of children. Diverse groups of children are being listened to and questions are being posed that, just a decade ago, would have been seen as too challenging or controversial for our youngest citizens. (Willow et al, 2004, p 90)

In consultation exercises associated with the introduction of children's databases the sample populations have tended to be small and predominantly involve young people who have a relatively well-developed acquaintanceship with welfare services, with few younger children present. This is quite predictable, since youth workers and others in contact with older children are often used to recruit consultees. Focus groups predominate as the method of choice, and this seems sensible given the need to explore, tease out, and give people a chance to consider and discuss the matter. Within this approach, most of the consultation processes involve the use of scenarios – 'this is the sort of situation you'd be in, what d'you think the issues might be for you in it?'. Those consulted evidently find the consideration of practical situations a congenial way to consider some of the implications. However, there are some disadvantages. The *overall* frame is generally the firm property of those sponsoring the consultation – so it is not really an equal conversation and it lacks a certain transparency. In the findings (a number of the relevant studies are summarised in DfES, 2004a, 2004b, 2006), the children involved suggest many caveats ('it all depends …'); these caveats have not been sufficiently listened to, and so the findings should not be taken to be as reassuring to policy makers as they have been.

With their hedged responses and nuanced awareness, it seems that children and young people offered insights that were thought-provoking, if perhaps unsettling, to those who had a major information sharing programme to deliver. It was plain that children were able and willing to engage with this subject, wanted their views to be heard, and were concerned to make *practical* suggestions. For example, the Healthy Respect Scottish national pathfinder project on adolescent sexual health talked with school-age students at some depth about privacy in the context of sexual health services, and about their expectations of different professionals, and the gist of their suggestions is typical:

- Tell us what you're up to – and check before sharing!
- Do some practical things to help in this:
    - leaflets to explain our rights
    - explain the ground rules clearly to new arrivals
    - write up your ground rules and give us a copy
- Make sure we know how to complain, if an adult breaks these ground rules
- We do understand that different staff may have to work differently with confidentiality – but it helps if you're clear about this. (Morrison and McCulloch, 2003)

The salience of context for children in evaluating the sensitivity of information and its disclosure was striking. For example, they appeared aware of the nuanced sensitivity of basic information like address, school and professional involvements. This makes one wonder about the apparent complacency reported by the Department for Education and Skills (DfES) (DfES, 2004a, 2004b; Wilson, 2006). Alongside this appreciation of nuance, children often lacked awareness and confidence in the organisational ramifications of information handling (Hill and Morton, 2003). This makes trust, based on familiarity with information receivers and givers, operating on the basis of consent, very significant. These factors have been consistently highlighted as the primary conditions of support for information sharing (Barnardos, 2003; CIS, 2005; Morgan, 2006). Some children were more assertive over the mechanics, being quite specific about wanting to control precisely what, how much and with whom information is shared. Finally, they adhered to practicality almost throughout. The likely practical outcome was crucial to whether or not children and young people supported sharing. In general, sharing was all right so long as good things happened on the basis of it.

In my experience of the process and practice of information sharing consultation, it seemed that those involved mean well (Willow et al, 2004) and are aware both that it has to be worked at and that they are not always as successful as they might hope (Cleaver et al, 2004a). There is plenty of exhortation to develop a participative approach (Cleaver et al, 2004b, Toolkit). But this is time-consuming to do, and is difficult to dovetail with one's other project activities, unless the phasing for the rest of the project is built around it. Projects tend to be shaped by groups of policy makers and their advisers, and children tend not to be involved at this early point. Once a project is moulded as either information technology or participation (and the two have not tended to mix well together), it is very difficult later to reinsert elements of either into the other. There are nonetheless some signs of learning from experience, which need to be welcomed.

The official vision is summarised in the DfES Engagement Plan for the Information Sharing Index (DfES, 2006). But perhaps this is all a bit late. The document makes it quite clear that the Index concept itself is not up for discussion – it is now a given. This is rather worrying given general experiences of such things as the difference between the design and actual use of systems, and function-creep over time (Anderson et al, 2006).

So, being child centred has not necessarily included really listening to children about their views on how their personal information is handled, or so it has been argued (Wilson, 2006). Perhaps we should not be too surprised, given opposing policy thrusts: liberty against protection, invigilation (howsoever benevolent) against empowerment. These thrusts reflect our contradictory attitudes towards children, who are perceived simultaneously as threatened and threatening, and our ambiguous attitude to what response the state should make. Policy errs on the side of overprotection, embodying traditional constructs of children as 'at risk' and 'in need', and disregarding shifts in, for example, the theoretical model of children's competencies (Willow et al, 2004).

Public discourse on children's databases has been contentious. Reading the volumes of published materials (the Lords debates are a good case in point, for example Hansard, 2004) one is left with the impression of little fruitful dialogue between the opposing points of view. Kelley's comment on the outcome of consultation on non-consensual information sharing is worth quoting in full for tone as well as substance:

> This is not an example of children and young people putting forward an idea [on potential criteria for information sharing without consent] that is unrealistic or unworkable. Their consensus view is similar to the current legal position, as were those two views expressed by a wide range of adult stakeholders including the major UK children's charities, rights based organisations, and the government's own Information Commissioner, who described the proposed databases as a policy indicative of a state 'sleepwalking into a surveillance society'.
>
> How much impact did these views have on the developing policy? The simple answer is none: S12 of the Children Act 2004 created a power for the secretary of state to require all children's services authorities to set up databases with the same structure and function as those described in Every Child Matters. (Kelley, 2006, p 39)

On balance I am left with an impression that it might have helped to be more transparent about the privacy issues. Here the notion of some form of consistently applicable framework for a series of conversations comes to mind. In Scotland the children's services information sharing programme commissioned a privacy research project (Raab et al, 2004), which was intended to help officials work out a balance between the potentially conflicting requirements of privacy and protection of the child. The research project assessed the feasibility of doing a Privacy Impact Assessment (PIA). A PIA comprises self-administered procedures and techniques, rather than some artefact to which one would delegate handling of privacy issues. The potential contribution of this is discussed later in the chapter.

Framing the discourse

Through my experience of project management I have learnt about how much time needs to be spent on framing and reframing, if people are to act within a general shared context rather than wait to be told exactly what to do. Working with the frame used by any stakeholder – perhaps trying to help them shift from one to another – is crucial for creative engagement.

Faced with empirical evidence that quite sane people were capable both of quite different understandings of the same problem, and of varying their own understanding depending on their appreciation of the context they saw themselves as in, researchers in a Performance and Innovation Unit (PIU) project were struck by the explanatory power of the idea of a 'frame' (of reference) (6, 2005). This theoretical construct has a respectable pedigree within the sociology of knowledge. Applied to privacy and information sharing, it has been termed 'privacy pragmatism' (PIU, 2002) (see Box 9.1).

Box 9.1: Privacy pragmatism

- People consider privacy within the context of their service experience. Besides the working out of this in a series of hypothetical scenarios discussed by the PIU focus groups (6, 2002), one can also see it in some of the contemporaneous early work on electronic health records (ERDIP) where the concept of a 'footprint of trust' (Singleton, 2002) was articulated around key transition points on patient pathways and equivalent welfare careers (Corbett, 2002). Of course, this may not necessarily apply literally to children – perhaps because they have not yet had to trade privacy for services. On the other hand, they will perhaps be aware of trading personal confidences (Lenhart and Madden, 2007), so the all-important notion of trade can still be explanatory.
- Within this paradigm, trade-offs are made between privacy and service provision – and people are well aware of this. They just have tended not to articulate it, although the recent TrustGuide research begins to do this (Lacohee et al, 2006).
- Service users' experience of practitioners crucially informs the level (Duffy et al, 2003) and type (6 et al, 1998) of trust in the service organisation concerned.

In the consultations with children and young people described earlier (DfES, 2004a, 2004b, 2006), these children and young people were offered scenarios that the policy makers thought were relevant. The various (although limited in range) frames of reference that are observable behind the scenarios are perfectly worthy in themselves. However, the frames were not an adequate basis on which to build information systems that are intended to apply to whole populations. Moreover, besides the question of whether the frames were sufficient to cater for envisaged future trends in the handling of personal information within children's *services*, there is also a broader question of their sufficiency within the *lives* of early 21st-century children.

Cultures of information sharing

Information sharing technology stands to be used to support sharing across different service domains with quite different sharing cultures and dynamics. For example, as between the worlds of health and social care on the one hand, and crime reduction and public protection on the other, key contrasts have been characterised as shown in Table 9.1 (6 et al, 2005b).

Differences in sharing practices are seen as reflecting general patterns of organisational accountability and culture rather than any confidentiality-specific issues. For example, 6 and Bellamy (2005) saw the culture of 'emergency as the norm', which encouraged looser sharing practice, as bearing more on crime contexts than health and social care. Also, clients' scrutiny of their own records was seen as a more

Table 9.1: Contrasts between information sharing in health and social care, and crime reduction domains

Health and social care	Crime reduction and public protection
• More sharing within teams but more protection of client data from others	• More diversity of sharing patterns • More pooling of data and shared access to databases
• Tighter interpretation of 'need to know'	• More explicit negotiation of appropriate sharing
• More awareness of clients' rights even at risk to staff and public	• Greater uncertainty about data protection and individual rights
	• Stronger assertion of duty to prevent risk to public, even when generalised and remote

legitimate activity in health and social care than for clients suspected or convicted of a crime.

The comparison of information sharing cultures across domains can be applied to children's information via the FIPR analysis, noted above, of the way principles first applied to the narrower field of child protection have been extended to the broader field of all children in need. Indeed, it has been suggested that this coverage stands to be extended a good deal further, to the mass of all 11 million children. These are children of 'people like us', rather than just 'them' – children needing special protection. Other than the Identity Project (LSE Information Systems and Innovation Group), the focus of most current discussion from this perspective has been the Information Sharing Index.

At this point the noticeable institutional and policy distinctions between children's welfare services and mainstream education, which involves children's aspirations to a much greater degree, come into view. Once we begin to consider handling data about aspirations, such as one might see in holdings on personal learning plans for all children, and not just needs and services, then the frame of reference jumps bodily sideways. Even the Information Commissioner's Office might find the ground shifting slightly under its feet. In England, the Digital Strategy for Education (DfES, 2005) refers to a 'personal learning space' for all pupils. In Scotland, one can find a detailed sketch of how a 'home page for every pupil' available via GLOW (formerly Scottish Schools Digital Network) (Davitt, 2006) is envisaged as supporting pupils and parents alike. Data on achievements and aspirations might seem non-controversial at first sight, but are arguably subject to similar levels of contingency as the demographic and address data discussed above.

Digital information and the lives of early 21st-century children

What sort of digital world is developing around our children? Let us look at just a few envisaged future trends.

The idea of a 'learning space' or anything more than a very basic home page is difficult to separate from one of the fastest-growing trends in all this: interactivity and the growth of user-generated electronic content – not just commenting on an assessment someone else has framed, but using your own plan, blog or YouTube video upload to reflect on what you want to do next with your life and celebrate all manner of things you have been involved with. Much of this is loosely gathered under what is known as 'Web 2.0', and it is a sign of how significant this may be that the BBC's online strategy for the next five years puts it at its core (Thompson, 2006; Loosemore, 2007). One should not presume that *everyone* is uploading their party photos to Flickr (Gibson, 2005) and the like. But the trend curve is still pretty steep (ScotEdublogs, 2006).

Of course, speaking and publishing, commenting and tagging (Marlow et al, 2006) say something about the speaker as well as the subject under discussion, and the levels of self-disclosure among young people have been commented on (boyd, 2006b). In some cases, sharing personal information has gone well beyond abstract impersonal data (CAPA, 2007). On the other hand, most participants' information sharing activity with 'friends' and contacts on social networking sites (such as Bebo, Facebook, MySpace; see Bowley, 2006; Noguchi, 2006) is more productively considered as part of 'exploring personal digital identity'. Sharing behaviour in Facebook has been characterised as that which tends to take place within communities of kindred spirits, and perhaps the value perceived by the young in (a sort of inverted) privacy enhancement via digital technologies is related to this. The findings from the UK Children Go Online study (Livingston and Bober, 2005) suggested that among the things a proportion of children appreciated about going online was relative privacy there from their parents and families (Slatalla, 2007).

The discourse is taking place within a context where technology has clearly enabled a shift away from a dichotomy between public and private (public/published versus private/one-to-one communication) to a gradient (when a mass email finally becomes 'publishing'; Davies, 2005). A connecting thread through most of these aspects of digital life for 21st-century children is the development of early (and as yet rather primitive) forms of support for 'faceted identity' management. Boyd has discussed these forms in terms of overlapping social networks (boyd, 2002, 2006a; Lenhart and Madden, 2007), and the way young people learn to handle the necessary linkages, but arguably, faceted identity has a chronological element too (Wallon, quoted in Alvergnat, 2001).

Finally, we should be aware of the general growth in digital learning and associated literacies. This is associated with the notion of children as 'digital natives'. It is easy enough to draft cheerful and thoroughly comforting scenarios and imagine that a Good Fairy will magically implement them tomorrow. Is it sensible, or rather conservative, to envisage the development of this into a *universal* experience as a lengthy process (Owen, 2004)? The landmark research report from the London School of Economics and Political Science (Livingstone et al, 2004) was relatively conservative on levels of user-generated content as compared with browsing, although one should remember its relative age in what is a pretty fast-moving domain. Where they are already involved and have access, the depth of children and young people's skills, and their developing acquaintanceship with key constructs such as cyber trust (Lacohee et al, 2006), are racing ahead (Green and Hannon, 2007: Sarson, 2007). While the digital divide still needs to be borne firmly in mind here just as much as generally, what is clear is that major policy, institutional and technological resources have been committed (Davitt, 2006).

Reconsidering frames

How can we bridge from the limited group currently the target of our consultation efforts – children with needs – to working with the skills of the whole child population? I suggest that we need three things: some theory; a medium within which to apply it; and a practical context within which to work.

For theoretical underpinnings, I suggest that privacy pragmatism as applied to information sharing could be adapted to suit the wider context. A version (see Table 9.2) of 6's grid of frames (6, 2002) could support identification of most children's relation to services.

For a medium or conduit for applying insights that one might wish to explore, I would suggest trying out a PIA. The 'PIA is ideally a project self-assessment tool, with external review – not: an audit, an obstacle, a legal compliance tool, a checklist, a one-time assessment' (Raab, 2004). It is a form of investigative instrument – a mechanism for organising discourse about the privacy impacts of proposed information handling, and assessing the balance between the proposed sharing and implications for privacy. Besides its organising capability it is also a conversation script – although one which allows judicious ad-libbing – and a framework that the various stakeholders in transparent discourse can engage with.

One of the advantages of an instrument like this is that once a template for its application to any data domain has been created, the assessment can be rerun at a number of organisational levels and on a number of occasions. This enables various groups of stakeholders to have their own conversations, or review them against what they thought earlier, and come to their own appreciations of the implications for their own privacy – rather than simply being players in someone else's game entirely.

Finally, for a practical context for privacy discourse, I suggest we consider 'personal learning planning' (PLP). PLP is a significant mechanism for the application of Assessment for Learning within

Table 9.2: Children's contexts and experiences

	Children's contexts	
Children's use of public services	*Largely aspirational*	*Less purely aspirational, also involving a good dose of remediation*
...Occasional, relatively inexperienced...	Primary school students, just getting an idea of where they are in their social and educational world	eg Not getting on very well at (secondary school), in contact with a variety of 'support' services (which they do not always experience as very 'supportive'. [tend both to under- and overestimate extent of data sharing; can be either frustrated or suspicious; want safeguards]
...or frequent, experienced...	eg Doing well in (secondary and/or tertiary) education, in contact with a number of aspiration-oriented provision (gapyear. com etc). Maybe have a Bebo/MySpace/Facebook account. [tend to under-estimate the extent of data sharing, and to find this low level of sharing frustrating: see lack of data sharing as incompetent, but want clear safeguards on data sharing]	eg Children in residential care, and/or involved with various elements of youth justice system. [tend to be resentful, and to a fatalistic over-estimation of extent of data sharing; see data sharing as malevolent, have little faith that safeguards will be respected]

Note: Sentences in [ ]s are direct quotes from the original.

Source: Adapted from 6 (2002)

Scottish primary and secondary education, and Assessment for Learning is itself a cornerstone of policy and practice across Scotland (LTS, 2005; SEED, 2005). PLP involves dialogue between children, parents and teachers. This dialogue focuses on what the child is going to be learning, and how those involved will know whether achievements and progress have been made. It also encompasses planning together for the next steps. The benefits conferred are seen as enabling children to develop 'greater responsibility for their own learning; improved confidence and self-esteem; a greater sense of involvement in planning for their own future' (SEED, 2006, p 5).

Local experience underpins my belief that personal learning planning can be used as the key cross-over point between needs-based and mass privacy concerns. In the latter days of work on the Integrated Assessment Framework, it became evident that it was conceptually quite possible to envisage a 'Single Plan' for children that an individual would take with him (or her) throughout childhood. The title, characteristics and associated processes of the plan would evolve with the individual's context, needs and circumstances, but it would work within an integrated framework, across all school-age students. At the time of writing, perhaps this concept remains a hard one to grasp for those involved in either schools or children and families service settings. However, along with being a universal activity in its own right, personal learning planning can be either the core of, or a significant building block within, the entire range of plans currently applicable to the much smaller groups of children with more appreciable needs. A child health profile could contribute to personal learning planning. An Individual Education Plan (IEP); a Comprehensive Support Plan (CSP); care planning built on a social work needs assessment, and within a Single Assessment Record and Plan (SARP) collated for all those children referred to the Children's Hearing system – all these can be built on in personal learning planning. With its other pointers towards the wider, social, personal (perhaps 'extra-curricular') elements within the lives of children, here is where personal learning planning offers a fruitful context for the beginnings of a properly rounded social discourse about privacy and public sphere information on our young citizens.

In consultation processes any conversation piece can be a useful support for collective endeavour. But it is also useful to have a framework that can be endlessly reused, and moved in a variety of directions given the different takes that different children and other actors will have. Each must have the time to engage with conversation pieces, and develop their own thinking (and associated literacies) and point of view in their own time. Besides conversation pieces, better training in consultation and relevant support for practitioners would not go amiss. But is 'better consultation' enough? Various proposals have been set out for public services that really listen to their users, and handle personal information appropriately in support of a radical approach that is closer to participation than consultation. These proposals are all rooted in what their authors see as 'what works socially'. This is crucial. Without this, technological sufficiency is simply insufficient.

Any sustainable framework will need to operate at a number of levels: high-level goals (the equivalents of mission statements) through to concepts that individuals deploy in handling themselves in social contexts. So, at one level, we need to try harder at children's involvement in policy formulation. If we are not to be cynical about consultation, we need to *listen* to what children say, and do something on the basis of it. To help make this shift, we need to aim to incorporate our discourse within mainstream activities rather than purely mainstream *consultation*. And we need to develop better contexts for the individual working out of solutions and acquisition of skills.

Acknowledgements

This piece has been informed by the pleasure of working with so many colleagues that it would be almost invidious to identify any individuals. But I would like to give special thanks to Marina Copping for her generous offer of the opportunity to consider this topic, and to Tamsyn Wilson for the welcome spur – and indeed the original means – to get on and do something about it.

References

6, P. (2002) *Strategies for Reassurance: Public Concerns about Privacy and Data-Sharing in Government*, London: Performance Innovation Unit, Cabinet Office, www.cabinetoffice.gov.uk/strategy/downloads/su/privacy/downloads/piu-data.pdf

6, P. (2005) 'What's in a frame? Social organisation, risk perception, and the sociology of knowledge', *Journal of Risk Research*, vol 8, no 2, pp 91-118.

6, P. and Bellamy, C. (2005) 'Information-sharing and confidentiality: local settlements?', Presentation to policy-makers' seminar, Edinburgh, 24 October.

6, P., Bellamy, C. and Raab, C. (2004) 'Data-sharing and confidentiality: spurs, barriers and theories', Paper presented to the Policy Studies Association Conference, University of Lincoln, 5-8 April.

6, P., Laskey, K. and Fletcher, A. (1998) *The Future of Privacy: Vol 2, Public Trust and the Use of Private Information*, London: Demos.

6, P., Raab, C. and Bellamy, C. (2005a) 'Joined-up government and privacy in the United Kingdom: managing tensions between data protection and social policy. Part I', *Public Administration*, vol 83, no 1, pp 111-33.

6, P., Warren, A., Bellamy, C., Raab, C. and Heeney, C. (2005b) 'The governance of information-sharing in networked public management', Paper presented at the 8th Public Management Research Conference, School of Policy, Plannng and Development, University of California, 29 September-1 October.

Alvergnat, C. (2001) *Internet et la Collecte de Données Personnelles auprès des Mineurs*, Paris: Commission Nationale de l'Informatique et des Libertés (CNIL), www.cnil.fr/index.php?id=94

Anderson, R., Brown, I., Clayton, R., Dowty, T., Korff, D. and Munro, E. (2006) *Children's Databases – Safety and Privacy. A Report for the Information Commissioner*, Foundation for Information Policy Research, www.ico.gov.uk/upload/documents/library/data_protection/detailed_specialist_guides/ico_issues_paper_protecting_childrens_personal_information.pdf

Barnardos (2003) *Every Child Matters: Response from Children, Young People and Families who use Barnardos Services*, Ilford: Barnardos.

Bellamy, C., 6, P. and Raab, C. (2005) 'Joined-up government and privacy in the United Kingdom: managing tensions between data protection and social policy. Part II', *Public Administration*, vol 83, no 2, pp 393-415.

Bowley, G. (2006) 'The high priestess of internet friendship', *Financial Times*, 27 October, www.ft.com/cms/s/59ab33da-64c4-11db-90fd-0000779e2340.html

boyd, d. (2002) 'Faceted id/entity: managing representation in a digital world', Masters thesis, Massachusetts Institute of Technology, Cambridge, MA, www.danah.org/papers/Thesis.FacetedIdentity.pdf

boyd, d. (2006a) 'Identity production in a networked culture', AAAS paper, www.danah.org/papers/AAAS2006.html

boyd, d. (2006b) 'MySpace parental paranoia: study shows fear of MySpace predators is overblown', www.zephoria.org/thoughts/articles/2006/07/10/study_shows_fear.html

CAPA (Child Abuse Prevention Association) (2007) 'MySpace and internet safety', blog posting, www.childabuseprevention.org/blog/?p=14

CIS (Children in Scotland) (2005) *Report of Consultation Events with Children and Young People: Getting it Right for Every Child: Proposals for Action*, www.scotland.gov.uk/Publications/2006/03/13104913/0

Cleaver, H., Cleaver, D. and Woodhead, V. (2004b) *Information Sharing and Assessment: The Progress of 'Non-trailblazer' Local Authorities*, Research Report 566, London: DfES. [Related Toolkit for document development and examples from non-trailblazer authorities available via www.cleaver.uk.com/isa/ including 'Participation of Children, Young People and Families'.]

Cleaver, H., Barnes, J., Bliss, D. and Cleaver, D. (2004a) *Developing Information Sharing and Assessment Systems*, Research Report 597, London: DfES, www.dfes.gov.uk/research/programmeofresearch/projectinformation.cfm?projectid=14439&resultspage=1

Corbett, B. (2002) *Project 3 Consent & Confidentiality Deliverable: Part PO 3.1 (revised)*, Tees ERDIP Demonstrator Programme, Birmingham: NHS Information Authority.

Davies, W. (2005) *Modernising with Purpose: A Manifesto for a Digital Britain*, London: Institute for Public Policy Research, www.ippr.org.uk/publicationsandreports/publication.asp?id=297

Davitt, J. (2006) 'Scotland wakes up with a healthy GLOW', *Guardian Education*, http://education.guardian.co.uk/elearning/story/0,,1875257,00.html

DfES (Department for Education and Skills) (2004a) *Every Child Matters: Report of Consultation Meetings with Children and Young People*, London: HMSO.

DfES (2004b) *Every Child Matters: Analysis of Children and Young People's Responses to the Consultation Document*, London: HMSO.

DfES (2005) *Harnessing Technology: Transforming Learning and Children's Services*, London: HMSO. Summary available at www.dfes.gov.uk/publications/e-strategy/docs/e-strategysummary.pdf

DfES (2006) *The Information Sharing Index: Children, Young People and Families Have Their Say*, London: HMSO, www.everychildmatters.gov.uk/resources-and-practice/IG00155/

DH (Department of Health) (2000) *Framework for the Assessment of Children in Need and their Families*, www.dh.gov.uk/en/Publicationsandstatistics/Publications/PublicationsPolicyAndGuidance/DH_4003256

Duffy, B., Downing, P. and Skinner, G. (2003) *Exploring Trust in Public Institutions: Report for the Audit Commission*, MORI, www.ipsos-mori.com/publications/srireports/pdf/final.pdf

ESRC (Economic and Social Research Council) (2003-05) *Joined-Up Public Services: Data-Sharing and Privacy in Multi-Agency Working*, www.esrcsocietytoday.ac.uk/ESRCInfoCentre/ViewAwardPage.aspx?AwardId=2666

Gibson, O. (2005), 'Young blog their way to a publishing revolution', *The Guardian*, 7 October, http://technology.guardian.co.uk/news/story/0,16559,1586891,00.html

Green, H. and Hannon, C. (2007) *Their Space: Education for a Digital Generation*, Demos, www.demos.co.uk/publications/theirspace

Hansard (2004) *Children Bill (HL) 24.05.04*, www.publications.parliament.uk/pa/ld200304/ldhansrd/vo040524/text/40524-03.htm#40524-03_head2

Hill, M. and Morton, P. (2003) 'Promoting children's interest in health: an evaluation of the child health profile', *Children & Society*, vol 17, no 4, pp 291-304, http://search.ebscohost.com/login.aspx?direct=true&db=pbh&AN=10816421&site=ehost-live

Introna, L. D. (1997) 'Privacy and the computer: why we need privacy in the information society', *Metaphilosophy*, vol 28, no 3, pp 259-75.

Kelley, N. (2006) 'Children's involvement in policy formulation', *Children's Geographies*, vol 4, no 1, pp 37-44.

Lacohee, H., Crane, S. and Phippen, A. (2006) *TrustGuide: Final Report*, October, www.trustguide.org.uk/Trustguide_-_Final_Report.pdf

Lenhart, A. and Madden, M. (2007) *Teens, Privacy, and Online Networks: How Teens Manage their Online Identities and Personal Information in the Age of MySpace*, Pew/Internet and American Life Project, www.pewinternet.org/PPF/r/211/report_display.asp

Livingston, S. and Bober, M. (2005) *UK Children Go Online Final Report: Key Findings*, London: London School of Economics and Political Science, www.children-go-online.net/

Livingstone, S., Bober, M. and Helsper, E. (2004) *Active Participation or Just More Information? Young People's Take-Up of Opportunities to Act and Interact on the Internet*, London: London School of Economics and Political Science, www.children-go-online.net

Loosemore, T. (2007) 'How the BBC is embracing the find, share and play attitudes of the Web 2.0 community', Presentation to the JISC Conference, Birmingham, 13 March, www.jisc.ac.uk/events/2007/03/event_conf_0307/commentary_loosemore.aspx

LSE (London School of Economics and Political Science Information Systems and Innovation Group) 'The identity project', http://is2.lse.ac.uk/idcard/

LTS (Learning and Teaching Scotland) (2005) 'What is an AifL School?', www.ltscotland.org.uk/assess/aiflschool/index.asp

Marlow, C., Naaman, M., boyd, d. and Davis, M. (2006) 'Position paper, tagging, taxonomy, flickr, article, toread', Collaborative Web Tagging Workshop (at WWW 2006), Edinburgh, Scotland, 22 May, www.danah.org/papers/

Morgan, R. (2006) *Passing It On: Views of Children and Young People on the Government's Guidelines for Sharing Confidential Information about them*, London: Commission for Social Care Inspection (CSCI), www. rights4me.org/reportView.cfm?id=7&startRow=9

Morrison, C. and McCulloch, C. (2003) *A Report on a Study Exploring the Issue of Confidentiality in Young People's Sexual Health Services*, Healthy Respect Project, www.healthyrespect.org.uk/Phaseone.htm

Noguchi, Y. (2006) 'In teens world, MySpace is so last year', *Washington Post*, 29 October, www.washingtonpost.com/wp-dyn/content/article/2006/10/28/AR2006102800803.html

Owen, M. (2004) *The Myth of the Digital Native*, Bristol: Futurelab, www.futurelab.org.uk/resources/publications_reports_articles/web_articles/Web_Article561

PIU (Performance and Innovation Unit) (2002) *Privacy and Data-Sharing: The Way Forward For Public Services*, London: Prime Minister's Strategy Unit, www.cabinetoffice.gov.uk/strategy/work_areas/privacy/index.asp

Raab, C. (2004) 'Information sharing: the relevance of privacy impact assessment', Presentation to the Social Services Research Group meeting 'Assessing the needs of vulnerable children: information-sharing, systems ... and solutions?', Stirling, 15 November.

Raab, C., 6, P., Birch, A. and Copping, M. (2004) 'Information sharing for children at risk: impacts on privacy', Edinburgh, unpublished.

Sarson, R. (2007) 'The kids are alright online', *The Guardian*, 10 May, http://technology.guardian.co.uk/weekly/story/0,,2075529,00.html

ScotEdublogs (2006) *Rough Guide to Growth of ScotEdublogging*, http://scotedublogs.wikispaces.com/

SEED (Scottish Executive Education Department) (2005) *Information Sheet on Assessment is for Learning*, Edinburgh: Scottish Executive, www.scotland.gov.uk/Publications/2005/09/20105413/54156

SEED (2006) *Practical Advice for Parents on Personal Learning Planning*, Edinburgh: Scottish Executive, www.scotland.gov.uk/Publications/2006/04/19141445/0

SEHD (Scottish Executive Health Department) (2001) *Guidance on Single Shared Assessment of Community Care Needs*, Edinburgh: Scottish Executive, www.sehd.scot.nhs.uk/publications/DC20011129CCD8single.pdf

Singleton, P. (2002) *ERDIP Evaluation Project N5: Patient Consent & Confidentiality Study Report*, Cambridge: NHS Information Authority.

Slatalla, M. (2007) 'omg my mom joined facebook!!', *The New York Times*, 7 June, www.nytimes.com/2007/06/07/fashion/07Cyber.html?ex=1183176000&en=beaccde667fb1b41&ei=5070

Thompson, M. (2006) *Royal Television Society Baird Lecture: BBC 2.0: Why On Demand Changes Everything*, BBC, www.bbc.co.uk/pressoffice/speeches/stories/thompson_baird.shtml

Westin, A.F. (2003) 'Social and political dimensions of privacy', *Journal of Social Issues*, vol 59, no 2, pp 431-53.

Willow, C., Marchant, R., Kirby, P. and Neale, B. (2004) *Young Children's Citizenship: Ideas into Practice*, York: Joseph Rowntree Foundation, www.jrf.org.uk/bookshop/details.asp?pubID=625

Wilson, T. (2006) '"It's my information, kind of": the perspectives of children and young people on privacy and data sharing', MSc thesis, University of Edinburgh.

TEN

Working with adults with incapacity

Susan Hunter and Lisa Curtice

Overview

Adults with incapacity are people who lack capacity to take specific or all decisions. They include people with dementia, people with learning disabilities, people with severe acquired brain injury, people with severe mental illness and people with severe communication problems due to a physical condition, such as stroke. This chapter considers the issues as they may affect adults with learning disabilities.

For at least a decade, the direction of travel in policy and practice in the support of people with learning disabilities, underpinned by a rights–based approach, has been towards more individualised support with the person themselves having a greater say and more control over their lives (Great Britain Parliamentary Joint Committee on Human Rights, 2008). The voices and stories of individuals are at last beginning to be heard (Smith, 2006). Meanwhile, public service reform aims to achieve efficiencies in public service delivery and greater responsiveness to the citizen. The emerging legislative framework in Scotland is intended to enable people who lack capacity by providing authority for decisions to be made on their behalf, for example to enable them to receive necessary medical treatment. However, when implemented in a risk–averse culture, there are dangers that restrictions on the grounds of protecting rights may overpower practices that seek to maximise the contribution of people who need support to participate. These issues have particular resonance for people with learning disabilities who, historically, have been at risk of being perceived as lacking competence or even 'subhuman' and certainly different from other members of society, with fewer needs (Wolfensberger, 1969).

Not all adults with learning disabilities will lack capacity, although this distinction may easily become lost. Moreover, as issues of risk and safety have risen up the policy agenda, the term 'vulnerable adults' has also come into use. It denotes adults (as distinct from children) who may be at risk of harm and therefore are felt to require measures of protection. This term, like the term 'adults at risk', which has quickly superseded it, may also too easily be used to refer to all adults with learning disabilities, as distinct from those who have been assessed to be 'at risk' in some way. It is also a cross–cutting term that can be applied to a range of people such as older people as well as to those with learning disabilities. The authors reject these labels as relevant to all people with learning disabilities. Rather, we seek to explore how these changing perspectives, both in legislation and in practice, impact on the rights of people with learning disabilities and specifically on issues of data sharing and confidentiality.

Consideration of the issues of privacy and confidentiality of personal information for adults with incapacity is informed in this chapter by a number of values and principles. We start from the assumption that all people have rights, regardless of their capacities, and that their capacity to have a say and exercise control should be maximised. The test of any public intervention should be the benefit or harm that it is likely to incur for individuals.

While the chapter is based on the emerging legislative framework in Scotland, the issues it raises are applicable in a wider context.

Context

Public services in general now use the language of citizenship (Scottish Executive, 2006a). Policy concerning people with learning disabilities had adopted a citizenship framework (Scottish Executive, 2000a; Secretary of State for Health, 2001). The aspiration was that people with learning disabilities should have the same opportunities as other people, should be able to live an ordinary life and should not be subject to discrimination. There was recognition that a key right was the right to have a say in what happened in one's life and in the services one received. More recently, citizenship rights have been proposed as the basis for greater control by individuals over their support and the funding to which they are entitled (Duffy, 2006).

The fact that people with learning disabilities may need support in, for example, managing their home or making decisions should not and need not be a barrier to their exercising their rights, for example to hold a tenancy agreement. In particular, independent advocacy can support people to have their wishes and intentions listened to and acted on (Mitchell et al, 2006). However, because the Western view of citizenship emphasises individual responsibility and substitute decision making if necessary, the idea that a person can be supported to exercise their full rights and role can be unfamiliar to some. (Beamer and Brookes, 2001, provide a full discussion of the British Columbia provisions for supported decision making.) Being on a jury and voting are examples of situations in which having support or a proxy are not seen as acceptable.

For many people with learning disabilities citizenship rights in practice may prove to be conditional – on access to advocacy, on availability of resources, on choice of supports and on the extent to which their voice is heard in decisions that affect them. There remains a considerable gap between the aspirations of people with learning disabilities for a home of their own, relationships and employment and their daily experience (Curtice, 2006). In particular, the rights of those who most need the support of others in order to have choices or participate may be considered vulnerable. While there is good practice in enabling people to be supported with communication, decision making and choices in daily living, people who are unable to exercise their autonomy independently may find themselves excluded from opportunities for relationships, supported living or even basic access to facilities (Emerson, cited in Stalker, 1998, p 66). The question this raises is whether citizenship rights are a sufficient safeguard to ensure universal human rights. Beckett (2006) proposes that human rights should be at the heart of citizenship; only when everyone recognises their vulnerabilities, he contends, will citizenship be truly protective of everyone.

The developing legislative framework in Scotland seeks both to protect rights and to provide authority for decisions and interventions for people who lack capacity. The 2000 Adults with Incapacity (Scotland) Act provides for decisions to be made on behalf of adults aged 16 and over who are unable to make decisions for themselves. Crucially, however, and unlike the preceding legislation, it allows for a menu of interventions on the assumption that capacity cannot be considered an 'all or nothing' concept. It is based on the five principles set out in the Act (Part 1, section 1(2)–(4):

- that there must be benefit to the adult that cannot be achieved in any other way;
- that the intervention should be the least restrictive possible;
- that the person's present and past wishes should be ascertained as far as possible, including the provision of any communication support required;

- that the views of the person's nearest relative and primary carer should be taken into account;
- that the person's capacity should be maximised; and
- that someone else should only take decisions for the person that he (or she) are unable to take for himself.

Where incapacity is established, the courts may award guardianship to another person to act in the interests of the adult with incapacity.

Capacity is defined as having information and being able to come to a decision on the basis of it, not being under undue pressure, being able to communicate the decision with any necessary support and holding consistently to the decision. The decisions the Act is concerned with are those about money and property and about health and welfare. People may have capacity in one area but not in another; their capacity may change over time and not all adults with learning disabilities will lack capacity. The 2003 Mental Health (Care and Treatment) (Scotland) Act builds on the principles of the 2000 Adults with Incapacity (Scotland) Act but its concern is with people with a 'mental disorder'. It therefore (controversially) covers the interests of people with learning disabilities, whether or not they have capacity. The overlap between these Acts can be a source of confusion to individuals, families and practitioners. The English 2005 Mental Capacity Act (implementation date 2007), following the Scottish Act by several years, shares many of the same principles, but crucially incorporates provision for Independent Mental Capacity Advocate Services. This provision is similar to that found in the Scottish mental health legislation. Both legal frameworks leave room for interpretation, for example in the assessment of capacity, and implementation of the Acts occurs in a context where the appropriate balance between enablement and protection is contested.

The balance between empowerment and protection is at the heart of current debates about policies and practice that affect people with learning disabilities. Self-advocates argue that an undue emphasis on risk can lead to unacceptable restrictions on their lives and deprive them of chances to learn from failure like everyone else. The unintended consequences of legislation have also included perceived restrictions on professionals' authority to take action to provide services for people's benefit. The Scottish government has had to clarify legislation in order to avoid guardianship or intervention orders being sought under Part 6 of the 2000 Adults with Incapacity (Scotland) Act in all cases where an adult with capacity was being moved (for example into residential accommodation) even where the adult did not object and no one disagreed with the decision. Some legal opinions had contended that professionals in local authorities did not have the authority to intervene to prevent harm or to enhance life for someone who cannot consent for themselves. However, Patrick (2004) argued for a less restrictive position, despite the *Bournewood* judgment (*R v Bournewood Community and Mental Health NHS Trust, ex parte L* [1998] All ER 319) and considered that the 1968 Social Work (Scotland) Act provided the local authority with sufficient powers to enable it to provide a community care service to an adult with incapacity, depending on individual circumstances. In February 2007 a new section 13ZA was inserted into the 1968 Act by amendment at Stage 3 of the passage of the 2007 Adult Support and Protection (Scotland) Act to clarify that, where a local authority has assessed an adult as requiring a community care service but the adult is not capable of making decisions about the service, the local authority may take any steps that it considers necessary to help the adult benefit from the service. However, these steps must not be incompatible with the European Convention on Human Rights (ECHR) including Article 5 on deprivation of liberty. Updated guidance (Scottish Executive Justice Department, 2007) issued in March 2007 seeks to prevent any unnecessary legal barriers to adults with incapacity receiving the services they need by setting out how the local authority can identify when an intervention would amount to a 'deprivation of liberty' and an order would be required.

Technology and data use in public service planning

Across the public sector there are commitments to promote data sharing, to streamline the many and different requirements for data collection and to make that data a more effective tool for measuring the outcomes of public policy (Scottish Executive, 2006a, 2006b). These are in part a response to concerns voiced by practitioners about the burdens imposed by an over-complex regulatory framework. They also represent an aspiration by government to develop the capability to demonstrate the difference that public expenditure is making to the lives of individuals receiving services. However, while considerable progress has been made in developing the technical infrastructure, progress in data sharing between professionals and agencies has been slow and self-advocacy organisations and others have had serious concerns. The two central issues are whether it is stigmatising to collect information about certain groups because of their impairment status and the legitimacy of the use of personal data for purposes other than direct service provision.

The review of services for people with learning disabilities, *The Same as You?* (Scottish Executive, 2000a), recommended that registers of people with learning disabilities should be set up in each area to provide better data for planning. The impetus for this recommendation came from the realisation that the actual numbers of such people in Scotland were unknown and therefore arguments for the need for resources and services had to be based on estimates. This 'invisibility' of disabled people in statistics is a global phenomenon. In the developing world there are few statistics of the numbers of disabled people despite the link between disability and economic disadvantage (Fujiura et al, 2005).

The proposal for separate databases about people with learning disabilities was seen by many, however, as incompatible with the general policy thrust that people with learning disabilities should be treated like everyone else, 'the same as you'. A further proposal to develop a national database of people with learning disabilities (and autistic spectrum disorders), in order to ensure comparable data nationally and influence the quality of locally collected data, has also aroused similar concerns. These include concerns about:

- stigma, because people with learning disabilities would be identified on the basis of their impairment;
- people with learning disabilities being singled out and subjected to greater invasions of privacy and surveillance than the rest of the population;
- information being used without people's knowledge in ways that might be to their detriment.

The historical experience of people with learning disabilities has led to considerable mistrust, both among self-advocates and practitioners, of the use of information about people without their knowledge. In particular, people with the label of 'challenging behaviour' may have been subjected to restrictions, rather than efforts being made to remove the cause of their distress (Emerson, 2001). In this context, description of impairments, measures of incapacity and records of needs may all become sensitive information because of the perceived risk that they may lead to restrictions on a person's life.

A project called eSAY has taken forward the development of the national database. Progress has been made in removing any disparity between data collection requirements for people with learning disabilities and other population groups. The eSAY project has become part of the overall development of national data standards, which should apply across all services. Core data items will apply to anyone who uses a service and particular data items relevant to certain population groups, such as people with learning disabilities, should therefore ultimately be collected across the public sector using common definitions. eSAY has developed the national data standards for learning disability (www. scotland.gov.uk/Topics/Government/DataStandardsAndeCare). However, concerns that the data items themselves are stigmatising have not been fully allayed and in the course of developing the dataset People First Scotland, the national self-advocacy group run by people with learning difficulties, withdrew from any involvement with the project.

In addition to developing standards so that data are consistent, there have also been national developments to safeguard the use of sensitive personal information in data systems. The national framework ensures that data are secure and that procedures take account of all relevant codes on confidentiality such as the 1998 Data Protection Act, the 1998 Human Rights Act and Scottish common law on confidentiality (Scottish Executive Data Standards and eCare Division, 2005). Consent is dealt with through local Information Sharing Protocols. Consent to share information must be agreed between agencies, but it is a local decision as to whether consent from the citizen is required for data that have been provided in the course of service delivery.

Thus, eSAY has become part of a much wider development in the public sector, which is seeking to improve the compatibility and capacity of IT systems, provide a legal framework to enable information sharing and improve the quality and relevance of data to improve public services. Rather than creating a separate database it aims to pool data that has been collected from routine service contacts within the framework of consent to share data that has been provided locally. All data are completely anonymised before being passed on to eSAY and there are many safeguards built into the system to prevent any identification of individuals. This approach means that people with learning disabilities are not being treated differently in terms of data collection and sharing. The data standards should be embedded in routine data that are collected in the course of service delivery. However, this more sustainable approach may also make it harder to show any immediate benefits from the system and means that the collection of data about people with learning disabilities has to compete with other information priorities at local level. There is no specific consent for data to be used in eSAY as this is now purely an anonymised aggregation of locally collected data. This is complex to explain and may make it harder to reassure people about the security of the data.

The eSAY project illustrates the potential conflict between the need for data that demonstrate the benefit of investment in services and the rights of individuals to 'have a say' about how information about them is used. While the legal frameworks and technical capabilities to share data safely must be developed, they are not a sufficient answer. Fujiura et al (2005) argue that there should be a shift in the type of data collected about disabled people. Rather than being impairment and deficit focused, data should be collected with the purpose of equalising opportunities and should consider the factors that relate to economic and social disadvantage. This reorientation of the content and use of data to address the multiple inequalities that disadvantage disabled people is much more likely to support public policies that seek to end discrimination than data that solely describe the prevalence of impairment (DRC, 2006; NHS National Services Scotland, 2007). The Disability Rights Commission argued that disability needs to be repositioned in public policy as a matter of 'equality, human rights and citizenship' (DRC, 2006, p 10). The test for information and data collection exercises will be the extent to which they contribute to this goal.

Data sharing in individual care planning

Barriers to information sharing are not confined to the collection of population-based statistics. Practitioners experience conflicts in decision making about when to share information, even in cases of assessment and direct service delivery. Some interpretations of the 1998 Data Protection Act contribute to a risk-averse culture in which professionals feel vulnerable if their disclosure should prove inappropriate. Professional culture also plays a part in whether a given professional may tend to the cautious protection of confidentiality (more common in the health service) or a greater readiness to share information (Richardson and Asthana, 2006).

The prolonged and appalling physical and sexual abuse of a woman with learning disabilities who had been receiving services from both social work and the National Health Service (NHS) in the Scottish Borders since childhood has led to fierce debates about how best to protect adults who are vulnerable. Just as not all adults with learning disabilities lack capacity, so not all are necessarily 'vulnerable adults'. However, professionals in health and social care need skills to identify circumstances that place people at risk of harm. The investigation into the harm suffered by this woman over several decades revealed that failures to share information were very significant in creating a situation in which no one had a full picture of what had happened and was happening (Mental Welfare Commission and Social Work Services Inspectorate, 2004).

Key issues in this case included poor practice in recording and above all in using information. Professionals seemed unwilling to exercise their responsibility to intervene and lacking in knowledge of the grounds on which they could do so. In fact, health and social work professionals were in possession of information for many years that should have led them to intervene to prevent further abuse, but they failed to do so. Information was poorly recorded and the information was not drawn together or used to assess risk. The person being abused was never interviewed alone and neither she nor another person who was vulnerable in the household had an independent advocate. These reports found that professional conduct had fallen short of the standards set by the Scottish Social Services Council Codes of Practice for social services workers, which require staff to 'promote the independence of service users while protecting them as far as possible from danger or harm'. A critical factor in the failure of services to protect this individual was the social workers' erroneous belief that they needed to have evidence that would meet standards of criminal proof before they had a right to intervene. They believed that they had no grounds to apply for guardianship to protect the person because allegations of abuse had been withdrawn. Social work and health services did not agree on the case for intervening and did not share information appropriately. The inquiry by the Social Work Services Inspectorate concluded that:

> This lack of any authoritative co-ordination, sharing and consideration of all the information held on each of the individuals and its interaction was a critical failure in the effective management of the case. (Social Work Services Inspectorate, 2004, p 9)

Following this case, pressure for new legislation to protect vulnerable adults has emerged. This proceeds from a concern that there may be people at risk of harm who are not covered by the incapacity or mental health legislation, and where powers may be needed to intervene for their protection. However, the power to intervene against the wishes of an adult who has capacity has been strongly contested by disability organisations who consider that this is a breach of human rights. At issue is the balance between the responsibility to protect from harm and the right to take risks. The 21st-century review of social work in Scotland (Scottish Executive, 2006b) has emphasised the need for practice and citizen leadership to ensure that services enable citizens to live full lives; under debate is how to develop safe practice that does not undermine aspirations for inclusion (Changing Lives User and Carer Forum, 2008).

Efforts to protect vulnerable adults may challenge the confidentiality regulations and practice of agencies and professions, as well as the behaviour of individual practitioners. Indeed, it has been argued that traditional professional codes of ethics and confidentiality based on one-to-one relationships are 'naive' and 'lack subtlety' in a modern world where the public is highly informed and services highly interactive. Hughes and Louw (2002) propose that (in the context of cognitive impairment) 'confidentiality is a myth it would be better to regard as a useful token of trust' (p 150).

The requirement for systems and practice to serve the citizen is more, not less, important for citizens who may be considered vulnerable. New powers would therefore only be part of the solution and should not be at the expense of individual rights. New legislation – the 2007 Adult Support and Protection (Scotland) Act – will create local multiagency protection committees that are intended to contribute to the development of a climate of trust and improved interagency procedures and working. The Codes of Practice will emphasise the importance of good assessment as part of professional practice. To date, progress on implementing Single Shared Assessment for any except older people has been patchy as has progress in data sharing through the Joint Future Agenda (Scottish Executive, 2000b). Multidisciplinary assessment, awareness of the preventive value of proactive data sharing within a framework of appropriate safeguards, acceptance of the professional responsibility to coordinate information and a willingness to listen in a safe environment to the voice of the person at risk and take his (or her) allegations seriously are all needed to protect vulnerable citizens.

Smart technology: possibilities and problems

The ready ability to share information, whether individual or systemic, has been transformed by advances in computer systems, but we now also possess the capability to increase support to vulnerable people in their own homes through the development of smart technology. This goes beyond the last generation of housing adaptations typically installed in supported housing for people with physical disabilities. Electronic technologies known as 'telecare' have been developed primarily to maintain older people in their homes for longer, with greater autonomy and less risk. Indeed, the Department of Health (2005, quoted in Bowes and McColgan, 2006) has set aside £80 million in grant monies to support these developments.

New models of telecare also bring concerns about intrusion of privacy and surveillance, possibly without consent; preoccupation with 'risk' and reinforcement of a medical model of care; and loss of focus on service models promoting inclusion as a policy objective. West Lothian Council in Scotland has been at the forefront in Europe of strategic service developments in telecare as part of a radical restructuring of its services for older people away from residential care (Bowes and McColgan, 2006). In addition to mainstreaming the basic service to older people over the age of 60, it has begun to make the resource available to a wider range of user groups including disabled adults.

Interestingly, there is scant discussion of capacity to consent in Bowes and McColgan's (2006) study, although people with dementia are beneficiaries of the augmented packages of care likely to include surveillance technology. The reader is left to conclude that the evident advantages of enhanced independence at home, informal carer support and cost-effectiveness outweigh other ethical considerations. As these electronic systems become increasingly incorporated into models of care for individuals who are vulnerable and lack capacity, we shall see the emergence of a debate about the nature of consent, resonating with the ethical, modernising agenda manifest in Hughes and Louw's (2002) discussion of the difficulties generated by legalistic interpretations of confidentiality.

Capacity and consent in research

In addition and closely related to issues of confidentiality in service provision, those of consent and control arise in research, particularly in respect of adults who may lack capacity to consent. Part 5 of the 2000 Adults with Incapacity (Scotland) Act deals with medical treatment or research. Participation in research can be authorised under certain conditions with adults who cannot give consent. The Code of Practice, which does not in itself have legal force but may have legal implications if not followed, sets out the position (Scottish Executive 2002, pp 32-3). The overriding principle is that similar research could not be conducted on adults who could give their consent. Further conditions are that:

- the research must either be of direct benefit to the individual or, exceptionally, benefit others with similar impairments;

- the person himself does not indicate an unwillingness to participate;
- the research involves little or no risk or discomfort;
- consent has been obtained from a person with relevant powers (for example, a guardian or welfare attorney with powers to consent to research participation or the adult's nearest relative); and
- the research has been approved by the Ethics Committee.

The legislation can therefore be seen as enabling, in so far as it provides for the possibility of proxy consent so that research can be authorised with adults who are deemed incapable of giving consent to research.

Nonetheless, the safeguards intended to prevent the exploitation of people who cannot give consent can lead to restrictions that make it very difficult to include them in research. While the overall principle of the Act, which of course applies equally to Part 5, is that incapacity is specific to the decision being made, that is, whether the person is able to consent to taking part in research, Part 5 adopts an impairment-based focus, referring to people with certain 'conditions'. There is an assumption that only people with the same impairment can (or should) benefit from research with people with significant impairments. This stance is contrary to the values of the disability movement and to many researchers in the field who would argue that the experiences of powerless and oppressed minorities will reveal issues about the way power structures and relationships operate throughout society. For example, the Fatal Accidents and Sudden Deaths Inquiry into the death of Jimmy Mauchland, a man with learning disabilities and complex needs, identified important failings in the way general hospitals care for people with complex needs. This had important lessons for wider patient care and demonstrated that evidence of the failure of care systems and practices to protect even the most vulnerable can be influential in bringing about change (Dunbar, 2003).

As well as the argument of public interest, there is an argument based in equity for weighting research practice to enabling, rather than restricting, the participation of people who have complex needs. It could be argued that, provided all the appropriate safeguards are in place, society should not deny to people with complex needs the possibility to participate in research if their experiences can benefit other people. People with the most profound impairments have usually not been included in research and as a result their experiences and the impact of treatments and services on them have not been taken into account. Improvements in services are often slowest for those with the greatest needs (Felce and Emerson, 2005). There is therefore an argument that it is a priority to improve the capacity of the research community to explore the experiences and evaluate the outcomes of services and treatments for everyone who receives these. Failing to record and take into account these experiences can be seen itself as a violation of identity and a suppression of 'hidden voices'. Facilitative approaches have been successfully developed that have made it possible to assist individuals to tell their stories (Booth, 1996; Atkinson and Walmsley, 1999; Goodley, 2000; Wilkinson, 2002; Fitzpatrick with Mitchell, 2006).

Research approaches based on trust and commitment to maximise the capacity of the individual may be difficult to express in ways that research ethics committees can recognise as good practice, particularly if they are only familiar with 'scientific' research designs. Hays et al (2003) describe how it took a full year and submissions to three multi-centre research ethics committees to gain approval to evaluate a course of cognitive behaviour therapy with men with learning disabilities and sexually abusive behaviour. In Scotland, Scott et al (2006) were delayed for 25 months in gaining approval to recruit children with learning disabilities for a research programme. They describe the burdens of the regulatory framework in terms of costs, time and paperwork, not only for themselves but also for the families concerned. These can be magnified in multidisciplinary contexts where there is not necessarily a consensus about good research practice.

Fundamental differences in values are exposed by the discussion about what constitutes good research practice with those who lack the capacity to consent to research. One position gives primacy to the protection of people from exploitation and seeks to restrict research with them, except where absolutely unavoidable. Another position questions the exclusion of some people from research that may be emancipatory and improve outcomes. It is arguable that complex regulatory systems do not necessarily provide an environment in which the most efficient and effective decisions about research practice and individual and public interest can be made.

Conclusion

Consideration of the issues affecting the ownership and use of personal data about people with learning disabilities highlights the contradictory imperatives in policies that seek to protect the interests of vulnerable adults while at the same time promoting their rights as citizens. Such contradictions create dilemmas for practitioners who may be unsure about what is the ethical or lawful approach in obtaining consent, sharing information, using potentially intrusive technology albeit for benign intent or undertaking research with people with profound disabilities whose needs we are least well informed about. This makes it highly unlikely, particularly in the present risk-averse climate of service organisations, that there will be any enthusiasm for taking the additional risk of sharing information across professional and agency boundaries. These ambiguities could be reduced if there were a much stronger commitment to share information with the vulnerable person and the data collected were clearly restricted to ensuring the well-being of that individual.

We are in a period of flux in understanding and practice as traditional conventions of professional ethics are brought into question and legal provisions are modernised to meet changing social structures and aspirations. Putting the person first may prove a robust approach to negotiating the maze of information sharing, just as it has proved a sure direction of travel for improving services and supports.

References

Atkinson, D. and Walmsley, J. (1999) 'Using autobiographical approaches with people with learning difficulties', *Disability & Society*, vol 14, no 2, pp 203-16.

Beamer, S. and Brookes, M. (2001) *Making Decisions: Best Practice and New Ideas for Supporting People with High Support Needs to Make Decisions*, London: VIA.

Beckett, A. (2006) *Citizenship and Vulnerability: Disability and Issues of Social and Political Engagement*, Basingstoke: Palgrave Macmillan.

Booth, T. (1996) 'Sounds of still voices: issues in the use of narrative methods in people who have learning difficulties', in L. Barton (ed) *Disability and Society: Emerging Issues and Insights*, London: Longman, pp 237-55.

Bowes, A. and McColgan, G. (2006) *Smart Technology and Community Care for Older People: Innovation in West Lothian, Scotland*, Edinburgh: Age Concern, Scotland.

Changing Lives User and Carer Forum (2008) *Principles and Standards of Citizen Leadership*, Edinburgh: Blackwell.

Curtice, L. (2006) *How is it Going? A Survey of the Views of People with Learning Disabilities in Scotland Today*, Glasgow: ENABLE Scotland and Scottish Consortium for Learning Disability.

DRC (Disability Rights Commission) (2006) *Putting Public Policy at the Heart of Disability in Scotland: Priorities for Action*, Stratford upon Avon: DRC.

Duffy, S. (2006) *Keys to Citizenship: A Guide to Getting Good Supports for People with Learning Disabilities* (2nd edition), Birkenhead: Paradigm.

Dunbar, I. (2003) 'Determination in the inquiry under the Fatal Accidents and Sudden Deaths Inquiry (Scotland) Act 1976 into the death of James Mauchland', Dundee: Sheriffdom of Tayside, Central and Fife, www.scotcourts.gov.uk/opinions/cb12_02.html

Emerson, E. (2001) *Challenging Behaviour: Analysis and Intervention in People with Severe Intellectual Disability* (2nd edition), Cambridge: Cambridge University Press.

Felce, D. and Emerson, E. (2005) 'Community living, outcomes and economies of scale', in R. Stancliffe and C. Lakin (eds) *Costs and Outcomes: Community Services for People with Intellectual Disabilities*, Baltimore, MD: Brookes.

Fitzpatrick, J. with Mitchell, J. (ed) (2006) *'I Don't Want to Miss a Thing': Stories of Regenerating Lives, from People Supported by the Thistle Foundation in Renfrew*, London: In Control Publications.

Fujiura, G. T., Park, H. J. and Rutkowski-Kmitta, V. (2005) 'Disability statistics in the developing world: a reflection on the meaning in our numbers', *Journal of Applied Research in Intellectual Disabilities*, vol 18, pp 295-304.

Goodley, D. (2000) *Self-advocacy in the Lives of People with Learning Difficulties: The Politics of Resilience*, Buckingham: Open University Press.

Great Britain Parliamentary Joint Committee on Human Rights (2008) *A Life Like Any Other? Human Rights of Adults with Learning Difficulties: Seventh Report of Session 2007-08*, London: The Stationery Office.

Hays, S.-J., Murphy, G. and Sinclair, N. (2003) 'Gaining ethical approval for research into sensitive topics: "two strikes and you're out?"', *British Journal of Learning Disabilities*, vol 31, no 4, pp 181-9.

Hughes, J. C. and Louw, S. J. (2002) 'Confidentiality and cognitive impairment: professional and philosophical ethics', *Age and Ageing*, vol 31, pp 147-50.

Mental Welfare Commission and Social Work Services Inspectorate (2004) *Investigations into Scottish Borders Council and NHS Borders Services for People with Learning Disabilities: Joint Statement from the Mental Welfare Commission and Social Work Services Inspectorate*, Edinburgh: HMSO, www.scotland.gov.uk/Publications/2004/05/19333/36719

Mitchell, D., Traustadottir, R., Chapman, R., Townson, L., Ingham, N. and Ledger, S. (eds) (2006) *Exploring Experiences of Advocacy by People with Learning Disabilities: Testimonies of Resistance*, London: Jessica Kingsley.

NHS National Services Scotland (2007) *Good Information for a Better Service? A Consultation with People with Learning Disabilities about Disclosing Personal Information*, A report by the Scottish Consortium for Learning Disability in collaboration with the Equality and Diversity Information programme, Glasgow: ISD Scotland.

Patrick, H. (2004) *Authorising Significant Interventions for Adults who Lack Capacity*, Edinburgh: Mental Welfare Commission.

Richardson, S. and Asthana, S. (2006) 'Inter-agency information sharing in health and social care services: the role of professional culture', *British Journal of Social Work*, vol 36, pp 657-69.

Scott, J.K., Wishart, J.G. and Bowyer, D.J. (2006) 'Do current consent and confidentiality requirements impede or enhance research with children with learning disabilities?', *Disability & Society*, vol 21, no 3, pp 273-87.

Scottish Executive (2000a) *The Same as You? Review of Services for People with Learning Disabilities*, Edinburgh: HMSO.

Scottish Executive (2000b) *Community Care, A Joint Future: Report of the Joint Future Group*, Edinburgh: Scottish Executive.

Scottish Executive (2002) *Adults with Incapacity (Scotland) Act 2000 Code of Practice for Persons Authorised to Carry Out Medical Treatment or Research under Part 5 of the Act*, Edinburgh: Scottish Executive.

Scottish Executive (2006a) *Transforming Public Services: The Next Phase of Reform*, Edinburgh: Blackwell's, www.scotland.gov.uk/Publications/2006/06/15110925/0

Scottish Executive (2006b) *Changing Lives:The Report of the 21st Century Social Work Review*, Edinburgh: Blackwell's, www.socialworkscotland.org.uk/resources/pub/ChangingLivesMainReport.pdf

Scottish Executive Data Standards and eCare Division (2005) *eCare Data Policy Statement*, Version 1.0, Edinburgh: Scottish Executive.

Scottish Executive Justice Department (2007) *Guidance for Local Authorities: Provision of Community Care Services to Adults with Incapacity*, CCD5/2007, Edinburgh: Scottish Executive Justice Department.

Secretary of State for Health (2001) *Valuing People: A New Strategy for Learning Disability for the 21st Century*, London: The Stationery Office.

Smith, N. (2006) '"I can make people listen"', *Community Care*, vol 1632, no 16, pp 20-6.

Social Work Services Inspectorate (2004) *Report of the Inspection of the Scottish Borders Council: Social Work Services for People Affected by Learning Disability*, Edinburgh: The Stationery Office.

Stalker, K. (1998) 'The exercise of choice by adults with intellectual disabilities: a literature review', *Journal of Applied Research in Intellectual Disabilities*, vol 11, no 1, pp 60-76.

Wilkinson, H. (ed) (2002) *The Perspectives of People with Dementia: Research Methods and Motivations*, London: Jessica Kingsley.

Wolfensberger, W. (1969) 'The origin and nature of institutional models', in R. Kugel and W. Wolfensberger (eds) *Changing Patterns in Residential Services for the Mentally Retarded*, Washington, DC: President's Committee on Mental Retardation.

ELEVEN

Working together? Sharing personal information in health and social care services

Val Baker

Introduction

In the 4th century BC Hippocrates made the following statement about the confidentiality of patient information:

> Whatsoever things I see or hear concerning the life of men, in my attendance on the sick or even therefrom, which ought not to be noised abroad, I will keep silence thereon, counting such things to be as sacred secrets. (Kennedy and Grubb, 1994, p 637)

If that were to be written today it might say:

> Whatever I see or hear in my attendance on the sick or even apart therefrom will be divulged to physicians, nurses, aides, anaesthetists, dieticians, physical therapists, admitting clerks, invoice clerks, discharge planners, record coders, medical records filing staff, chaplains, volunteers, performance evaluators, insurers, medical secretaries, public health officials, government officials, social workers and employers AND to whomever else requests them for whatever reason if appropriate. (Adapted from Givens, 1998, p 2)

This suggests the complexity of modern health systems and tests the assumption that our medical information is confidential. Add to that the need to share across health and social care service boundaries and it is understandable that the principle of 'private and confidential' becomes confused.

Professionals are expected to share appropriate information for the better health and care of patients and clients. That is clear. The rules of engagement, however, are a minefield of only partly understood jargon comprising a plethora of guidance policies and protocols. The introduction of fast electronic communication and integrated records has pushed the agenda of information sharing to the forefront. This chapter is about outlining some of the tensions this generates, and testing the definitions and use of the principles behind 'private' and 'confidential' in the implementation of manual and electronic shared data and information in the Scottish eCare programme.

Policy framework: Joint Future

The Scottish Executive published the report of the Joint Future Group in November 2000 (Scottish Executive, 2000a). This set in motion a range of formal processes in relation to joint working and information sharing between health and social care services, applicable in the first instance to older people and then to all adult groups. Since then, and in particular following high-profile child incident inquiries, a number of policies have been published in relation to sharing information about children, especially vulnerable children and those in need of care or protection. We need to remember, however, that any information about a vulnerable child inevitably includes, or at least reflects or refers to, information about an adult, either directly or indirectly.

The relevant policy and legislation in relation to joint working and information sharing includes:

- *Report of the Joint Future Group* (Scottish Executive, 2000a)
- 2000 Adults with Incapacity (Scotland) Act
- *Our National Health: A Plan for Action, A Plan for Change* (Scottish Executive, 2000b)
- *For Scotland's Children* (Scottish Executive, 2001) – 'a vision for integrated children's services'
- *'Its Everyone's Job to Make Sure I'm Alright'* – *Report of the Child Protection Audit and Review* (Scottish Executive, 2002)
- 2002 Community Care and Health (Scotland) Act
- *Partnership for Care: Scotland's Health White Paper* (Scottish Executive, 2003a)
- *Getting our Priorities Right: Good Practice Guidance for Working with Children and Families Affected by Substance Misuse* (Scottish Executive, 2003b)

- *Getting it Right for Every Child: Draft Children's Services (Scotland) Bill Consultation* (Scottish Executive, 2006b)

These formal documents propose a world where clinical and social care data flow freely between all those properly concerned with the care of an individual patient or client; where regulatory bodies and those such as NHS [National Health Service] National Services Scotland and local authority housing departments must be able to access a whole range of data to perform their functions; where joint working implies joint records; and where more and more emphasis is placed on information sharing. In such a world the issues of data security, data integrity and personal confidentiality become of crucial importance – not merely of theoretical or academic interest, but of intense practical relevance. If we do not safely resolve those issues and implement careful controls, much of the intent of information sharing will simply not work. Nevertheless, it is clear that major benefits in care delivery and efficiency savings could be made if information sharing is handled correctly.

'Joint Future' remains the lead policy on joint working between local authorities and the NHS in community care in Scotland. The principal aim is to provide faster access to better and more joined-up services through improved joint working. It expects joint partnerships to take holistic decisions on the management, financing and delivery of community care services for all groups.

Among the Joint Future report (Scottish Executive, 2000a) recommendations is implementation of a Single Shared Assessment (SSA). In England this is known as the Single Assessment Process (SAP). Partnership agencies in Scotland were expected to have SSA procedures in place for older people and for those with dementia by October 2001, and for all client groups by April 2002. Arrangements for SSA include specific proposals for the necessary sharing of information between agencies, by obtaining explicit client approval. The majority of Scottish Joint Future partnerships have implemented a form of SSA and many of those are electronic. Supporting implementation of SSA throughout Scotland there is an Information Sharing Protocol (ISP), which has been developed specifically for this purpose. Most partnership areas have developed a local version of a 'gold standard' suggested by the eCare programme (www.scotland.gov.uk/ecare).

The term 'Joint Future' was somewhat overshadowed when Community Health Partnerships (CHPs) came into being following the publication of the White Paper *Partnership for Care* (Scottish Executive, 2003a) and the ensuing legislation, the 2004 NHS Reform (Scotland) Act. The emphasis of implementation was on strong partnership links between health and social care, joint services and localised delivery of care led by frontline staff. In essence, CHPs could be seen as an extension of the fundamental principles behind the Joint Future work and so the data sharing programmes should continue and expand to encompass a wider range of joint services.

The Joint Future agenda has been complemented by a Scottish-wide programme of eCare initiatives. Outcomes and lessons learned from these programmes led to the development of a Scottish-wide review and during 2006 this formally became the Data Sharing and Standards Programme (Scottish Executive, 2006b). Each of the 14 Health Board areas in Scotland were invited to set up Data Sharing and Standards Partnerships consisting of Health Boards, local authorities, police and fire services as well as voluntary organisations. The Partnerships were given a set of priorities for local implementation, each of which was designed to increase local information sharing, especially in relation to child protection and adult SSAs.

Data sharing in the public sector

We cannot improve public services without first sharing data about service use and requirements. The Personal Data Directive of the European Parliament states that personal data is:

> any information relating to an identified or identifiable natural person (data subject); an identifiable person is one who can be identified, directly or indirectly, in particular reference to an identification number or to one or more factors specific to his physical, physiological, mental, economic, cultural or social identity. (European Parliament, 1995, Article 2, Definitions)

Data sharing is usually used to describe circumstances where public authorities routinely or on a foreseeable basis disclose personal data to other public authorities, either (i) for the purposes of the public authority or (ii) in a sharing arrangement where personal data are pooled and held in a new dataset to which a number of parties have access.

Purposes for sharing of personal information include:

- To deliver personal care and treatment.
- To improve quality of care and treatment.
- To monitor and protect public health.

- Manage and plan services.
- Audit joint services.
- Investigate complaints.
- Undertake risk management.

Personal data may also be disclosed by one public authority to another, or to a private authority, on a case-by-case basis. Such disclosures are neither routine nor foreseeable, but such instances are covered by local protocols.

The business information requirements of CHPs pertain to finance, the environment and aggregated resources. Collecting such data has not, so far, proven to be a major issue. It has not had the same political sensitivity as the sharing of personal data for patient and client care.

The need for agreements to govern the sharing of personal information has increased with the integration of health and social care, the development of electronic communication and the rights of individuals to respect for privacy. This has been recognised by organisations such as NHS Quality Improvement Scotland (QIS) that have developed a number of information governance standards that will help public services to support the information sharing agenda (see Box 11.1).

Box 11.1: Excerpt of information governance standards

A governance framework is in place which promotes ethical and lawful use of information in enhancing decision making to support and improve the quality of patient care, choice and services.

Patients are effectively informed about how their personal health information is collected and used, how to access their personal health information, and about their rights to determine how their personal information is shared.

Formal policies are in place to manage situations where patient consent to share information is withheld, and where disclosure of personal health information is required without consent.

Source: NHS Quality Improvement Scotland (2005, p 19)

Technology issues are relatively easy to solve given adequate funding and support. It is unifying the common processes, terminology, reporting, culture, multiagency agreements and the meeting of professional minds that poses the greatest challenges. However, understanding the rules of technology development helps us to grasp the issues facing community nurses and social care staff when sharing information. Those issues lie chiefly around security and confidentiality and the seemingly endless raft of legislative directives.

Understanding the principles and rules

Principles underpinning the rules and regulations include:

- openness and access;
- limiting collection;
- limiting use of information;
- storing and retaining appropriately;
- disclosure;
- secondary usage;
- informed consent;
- security of information;
- compliance with the rules;
- accountability.

The use of information about an individual is governed by statute law including the 1998 Data Protection Act and the 1998 Human Rights Act; the common law of confidentiality; official guidance; and professional standards and codes of conduct. Combined, these require users of data to be transparent, accountable and responsive to the needs of individuals (Scottish Executive, 2003c).

Statute law and regulations

1998 Data Protection Act

The 1998 Data Protection Act works in two ways, giving individuals certain rights while requiring those who record and use personal information on computer or manual records to be open about their use and to follow proper practices (see Box 11.2).

Box 11.2: Key principles of the 1998 Data Protection Act

Data should be:
- obtained and processed fairly and lawfully;
- obtained for one or more specified purposes;
- adequate, relevant and not excessive;
- accurate and where possible kept up to date;
- kept for no longer than necessary;
- processed in accordance with the rights of the data subject;
- stored using appropriate measures against accidental loss or destruction or damage to personal data.

Data should not be:
- transferred to a country outside the European Economic Area unless that country ensures an adequate level of protection for the rights and freedoms of data subjects.

The 1984 and 1998 Data Protection Acts embody the principles shown in Box 11.3.

Box 11.3: The principles of the Data Protection Acts

HORUS

Held securely and confidentially

Obtained fairly and efficiently

Recorded accurately and reliably

Used effectively and ethically

Shared appropriately and lawfully

2002 Freedom of Information (Scotland) Act (FOISA)

FOISA gives any individual anywhere in the world access to any recorded information held by Scottish public bodies. Exceptions include personal data covered by the 1998 Data Protection Act.

European Convention on Human Rights

Article 8 of the Convention holds that individuals have the right to respect for privacy and family life. There should be no interference with this right by a public authority unless it is in accordance with the law and necessary for the prevention of crime and disorder, for the protection of rights or morals, or for the protection of rights or freedoms of others.

2005 Re-use of Public Sector Information Regulations (SI 2005/1515)

These regulations came into force in July 2005. They do not change access provisions; rather they provide a framework for the re-use of information once access has been obtained. The aim is to unlock the value in public sector information and to allow the private sector to develop a range of value-added information services.

Official guidance

Caldicott

The Caldicott Report (DH, 1997) set in motion a process of continuous improvement in information handling. Sixteen principles were agreed by the committee and recommended to ensure that data handling was controlled. Caldicott principles were introduced into social care in 2001 (see Box 11.4).

> ### Box 11.4: Summary of Caldicott principles
>
> - Justify the purpose for using patient data.
> - Do not use patient-identifiable information unless it is absolutely necessary.
> - Use the minimum necessary patient-identifiable information.
> - Access to patient-identifiable information should be on a strict need-to-know basis.
> - Everyone should be aware of their responsibilities to maintain confidentiality.
> - Understand and comply with the law, in particular the 1998 Data Protection Act.

Public service guarantee

A public service guarantee for data handling is available for implementation by public bodies (Information Commissioner's Office, 2006). This sets out people's rights with regard to how their personal data is handled by public authorities and the standards they can expect public organisations to adhere to.

Committee on use of confidential personal information

The Healthcare Commission has produced a framework for obtaining, handling, use and disclosure of personal information for independent healthcare services (Commission for Healthcare Audit and Inspection, 2005).

Technical standards

Open Scotland Information Age Framework (OSIAF)

OSIAF is a key part of the Scottish Executive commitment to deliver world-class public services. It sets out standards and specifications used by the public sector and provides a framework for developing and approving interoperability specifications that support the delivery of electronic services (Scottish Executive, 2006c).

The eCare framework

This is the name given to a cohesive set of technology standards, architectures, infrastructure and software that enables multiagency information sharing within the public sector in Scotland (Scottish

Executive, 2006b). It enables with a single strategic approach secure electronic data sharing. The framework comprises data standards and policies, technical strategy, security, infrastructure and application standards and architectures. These include technical approaches for citizen identity management, citizen consent and legal disclosure for data sharing in a multiagency environment. The standards provide an agreed common view of the citizen that is applicable across all agencies that may need to share personal data.

Professional codes of conduct and practice

Professional and ethical codes of conduct include adherence to legislation and acknowledge an individual's right to privacy but enable the disclosure and sharing of information in appropriate circumstances. They are directed specifically at the profession for which the codes are written. Examples include:

- *European Standards on Confidentiality and Privacy in Healthcare* (McLelland, 2006)
- *Nursing and Midwifery Council Code of Professional Conduct* (Nursing and Midwifery Council, 2004)
- *Confidentiality: Protecting and Providing Information* (General Medical Council, 2000)
- *The Code of Ethics for Social Work* (BASW, 2002)
- *NHS Code of Practice on Protecting Patient Confidentiality* (Scottish Executive, 2003c)

Good practice notes are produced by numerous agencies in relation to specific activities, for example, taking photographs in schools, telephone marketing by political parties, providing personal information to a third party, individuals' rights of access to exam marks.

Dilemmas for professionals

Scenario

Mr Smith is 86 years old, lives alone and is visited twice a week by a care assistant who gives him a shower. He is about to go into hospital for a minor operation. Consider the range of people who need information – about the need for the operation, about a date and preparation for going to hospital for the operation, while he is in hospital, in preparation for discharge home, and finally when he gets home.

When should Mr Smith give consent?

What information is required by whom?

How is the information accessed?

Does Mr Smith know how many people have access to his information?

What if he does not consent to share information?

If all this information was on a computer, would you handle it differently to this information being on paper?

Almost every organisation that we deal with in our daily lives holds some personal information about us. Much will be confidential, some will be sensitive and much we do not want shared, certainly not without our knowledge. This is no different in health and social care than it is to a bank. Clearly, health and social care workers have to cope with what seem like conflicting objectives: the right to access information about individuals and the need for protection of personal data. They understand the need to share information where appropriate but are left to make professional judgements on what and when to share, the need for implicit or explicit consent, the need to know, exceptions to the rules, and ultimately to protect the privacy of the person in their professional care – a person who trusts them.

Confidentiality and privacy

Confidentiality pertains to the treatment of information that an individual has disclosed in a relationship of trust and with the expectation that it will not be divulged to others in ways that are inconsistent with the understanding of the original disclosure without permission. It has been defined by the International Standards Organisation (ISO, 2005) as 'ensuring that information is accessible only to those authorised to have access' and is one of the cornerstones of information security. Some simply define confidentiality as secrecy.

The core of confidentiality is about privacy, meaning that any information a person tells someone else about himself will be kept between the two of them. Keeping certain things confidential is an unspoken rule in a friendship. However, for health and social care professionals, confidentiality is based on adherence to the common and statute law, and here lies the heart of the confusion. Because the law allows for exceptions and professional judgement, in certain circumstances staff can be made to feel they have done wrong because they followed the expectations of the law.

Privacy has become one of the most important human rights issues of the modern age. At a time when computer-based technology gives government and private sector organisations the ability to conduct mass surveillance of populations, privacy is seen as a crucial safeguard for individual rights. As recently as November 2006 the Information Commissioner issued a press release in relation to the use of CCTV that sparked lively public debate on violation of privacy (Thomas, 2006). The increasing sophistication of computerised records, together with the capacity to collect, analyse and disseminate information, has introduced a sense of urgency for clear guidance and legislation (Davies, 2001).

Privacy is a fundamental requirement if health and social care staff are to maintain the trust of individuals who provide information in the provision of care. There are strong indications that public concerns about privacy and data use are becoming more marked. In 2002, the Performance and Innovation Unit published a report on privacy and data sharing (Cabinet Office Performance and Innovation Unit, 2002). It highlighted that to the public, crime prevention and improving education are the only issues thought to be more important than privacy. If organisations do not take this seriously there is a high chance of disengagement with the public, resulting in potential lack of information.

The Department of Constitutional Affairs was charged with responding to this report. The result is an action plan recommending that the move towards making more effective use of personal data would need to be accompanied by building public trust in the ways in which individuals' personal information was protected (DH, 2007). Recommendations include a review of policies and guidance, a reduction in legal requests for records and clearer guidance in relation to medical research.

Research from the Scottish Consumer Council (2005) highlighted that the public are concerned about data security. The NHS Information Authority commissioned a report (NHS Information Authority, 2002) on people's views on consent and confidentiality. In the main, people were more concerned about *who* used the information rather than *what* it was used for, and believed that only certain people should see certain parts of the information.

It would help privacy's case if one could show that members of the public value it highly. This would help in quantifying the benefits of good privacy protection. Unfortunately, most of the time (unless prompted, as in the Cabinet Office Performance and Innovation Unit's 2002 report) the public appears to view privacy with indifference, or fails to show any consistency. For example, people are often asked to trade their privacy in return for some benefit. It is commonplace to be asked for personal details in order to obtain access to 'free' services on Internet websites, or to qualify for loyalty cards or enter free draws. In practice, people often 'sell' their privacy at a cheap rate (Hawker, 2001).

Professional culture differences

There is also a difference in the understanding of confidentiality in practice between healthcare workers and social care workers. For healthcare workers the concept is fundamental. All health professionals are taught to protect information given by patients and it is central to the practitioner–patient relationship. Most health professionals believe that confidentiality is a cornerstone of their work and will breach it only in exceptional cases. But this position is increasingly under pressure.

Swain (2006) suggests that confidentiality as a concept derives from the patient–physician model, where the relationship is essentially dyadic, one to one. By contrast, much social work practice is non-dyadic. The social worker is always expected to consider the 'person in situation'. Personal information is not seen as the single concern and therefore information is collected about the environment that individuals find themselves in. Since it is not necessarily seen as personal it may not be understood to be confidential.

A theoretical review undertaken by 6 et al (2004) indicates that the heart of the data sharing issue is to be found in the relationship between the formal institutions of law and guidance on the one hand and the informal institutions of organisational and interorganisational functioning on the other. They suggest that handling of personal data in multiagency contexts involves unresolved tensions between what are widely perceived as conflicting values, which in turn highlights different perceptions of confidentiality.

Although community health services increasingly work within the 'situation', providing holistic care, there remains a strong sense of confidentiality in the relationship with an individual. If the patient wishes something kept from a relative, for instance, the community nurse will adhere to this wish except in specific circumstances.

Research shows (Richardson and Asthana, 2006) that this is less likely in social care circumstances owing to the nature of the organisation and service provision. It is said that social workers see information as being confidential within an organisation, rather than restricted to a particular individual (Moore, 2005). This is still not the view of medical and nursing staff, although it is shifting for district nurses and public health nurses. Richardson and Asthana (2006) showed that varying cultural attitudes have been researched many times and what seems clear is that there are differences in the way professionals work, how they define and tackle a problem, how individuals in their care are empowered, how the member of staff encompasses others in the solution and ultimately how the information is shared.

Joint working in itself suggests that 'person in situation' is the overriding principle and therefore sharing of information is the right and necessary thing to do. However, for the most part it relies on the consent of the individual providing that information – consent given with the assumption that the information will remain confidential to the partnership and for the purposes for which it was provided. Of course, there are exceptions where there are concerns about children and vulnerable adults and therefore a need to provide clear guidance for staff who are making the decision to override consent.

Given that organisational practice and cultural attitudes seem to have an influence on how data are shared, overall it seems unlikely that there is a shared understanding of confidentiality, of what needs to be shared and when.

Data sharing and informed consent

All professionals and agencies are required to keep confidential information given to them during the course of their work. Information given to professionals by their patients, clients or service users should not be shared with others without the person's permission, unless the safety of the person or other vulnerable people may otherwise be put at risk. Patient consent is generally required before information can be shared outwith the healthcare team. Most patients have not routinely, until now, been asked for consent to collect, share and reuse information. Nevertheless, it has been, and still is, common practice to ask for consent for specific treatments such as immunisation or anaesthesia. Practice on consent is changing.

Consent is required, however, for the collection of data for the Single Shared Assessment. This is consent relevant to that information at that point in time. Good practice is to fully inform the patient or client and therefore leaflets should be provided explaining why consent is required. Protocols and guidance must also be available for staff who may have to accept that some patients will withhold consent. There will be times when consent is not required and frontline workers must also be able to judge this appropriately.

Most of the information collected during a joint assessment will be reasonably straightforward. Clearly, there is a recurring overlap between health and social care information, especially in relation to provision of community care services. The priorities are to share demographic and recent care history, the latest assessment, outcome and care planned. Nevertheless, there are dilemmas facing community nursing and social care staff, which they may not realise from the outset of an assessment. The development of multiagency data stores, Single Shared Assessments, client indexes and joint care plans inevitably means that there is a large amount of information stored about an individual, which may be useful to others. Fair processing according to the 1998 Data Protection Act means that the information should only be used according to the purpose for which consent was given. The concept of 'need to know' at a point in the future is, understandably, ill defined. Without effective access control, privacy is at risk.

The temptation in any compilation of data, especially data which are as sensitive as those gathered by health and social care agencies, is to use them for other purposes. This happens and is called secondary use or reuse. Secondary use is, however, subject to regulation and this must also be explained to individuals. Discussions in relation to shared indexes of information, especially child information but also that relating to adult learning disability, mental health and other groups, have raised concerns about how such information will be used. It has the potential to affect future employment, access to state funding and the receipt of other services.

Research published by the Scottish Consumer Council (2005) showed that people in general do not know very much about how their personal information is stored and shared. They do support the increasing use of computers and recognise the benefits this can bring, but they are concerned about security and confidentiality and wish to be better informed. Research conducted by the Consumers Association (2003) confirmed this finding and also highlighted potential public concerns about the use of personal information.

Can we ensure that the informed consent provided at the point of information collection, with the understanding that the information is being obtained and shared for a specific purpose, will remain valid? For a hospital discharge involving community services, for instance, it is necessary to know when and how the individual is getting home, who his (or her) key workers are, whether equipment is needed, the level of support required, whether relatives are involved in care and so on. Information collected for this purpose, within the legitimate relationship of individual and expected service provider, is relatively clear cut. Individuals must be informed about the need to disclose information in order to provide high-quality care and they must believe that the information will be kept accurate and meaningful. They have a right to know what is being recorded and a right to access it themselves. They must be told what will happen to it and who is expected to have access to it and for what purpose.

Informed consent is important especially when data are compiled from a number of sources and used for multiple purposes. Best practice guidelines on review of consent are important but may be quite impractical for many services to implement, especially when shared access is enabled. Gaining consent at each point in the care pathway is certainly not practical and so the issue of when to get consent is not an easy one to solve. Consent forms need to be specific rather than all encompassing, but this is problematic and may be unworkable depending on when the consent is given. In addition to securing consent for specific purposes it will be necessary to specify the date of consent and a date for its review. People should not be asked to consent on unlimited timeframes.

High-profile cases, in the main relating to children (such as Climbié: Laming, 2003; and Ness: O'Brien et al, 2003) continue to identify inadequate information sharing as a contributing factor in the death of individuals being cared for by more than one agency. This places pressure on staff to share information without due consideration to organisational structure differences, variation in understanding of the terms of confidentiality and privacy, different language (client is a patient is an individual is a customer) and professional ethics. Balanced against the need to protect the privacy of the service users and the need to share information to deliver a service the whole issue becomes wonderfully complex.

In practical decision-making contexts there are tensions and conflicts between privacy and data sharing and between running opposing risks: false negative judgement errors (no action taken, but ought to have been taken if information had been shared); and false positive judgement errors (action taken but ought not to have been taken if privacy had been respected). Sometimes there will be adverse consequences of judgement errors. The current shift is towards intolerance of false negative judgement errors and preference for action even if false positive judgements are made (Bellamy et al, 2005).

Breaking confidentiality: ambiguous guidance

Decisions about when to involve other agencies and when to break confidentiality are difficult and complex. The Information Commissioner's Office (2006) called for public authorities to be encouraged to use and share data properly and not assume that all personal information can be shared. What does this mean? It may mean practitioners asking questions such as: Do I know something that may be useful for others to know? Is this information essential in providing the service? Who else is likely to see this information? Does the individual wish it to remain confidential? Do I have a right to share it without consent? Sharing of information is most challenging in sensitive cases such as sexual health, teenage pregnancy and childcare.

Much information can be shared within the guidance that exists. However, there appears to be confusion in the interpretation of the 1998 Data Protection Act and its relationship with the common duty law of confidentiality and other legislation such as the 1998 Human Rights Act, the 2001 Health and Social Care Act and information sharing legislation. Confusion is compounded by various regional and local guidance, professional guidance and protocols.

What actually happens? Is information kept confidential? How many get to see it? How secure is it? Is it well understood or misinterpreted? How much sharing is essential? Is it enough to share name, address and a few key data items? How will the data be handled over time? Will files be destroyed when no longer needed? What is the risk of developing a large-scale database, and might it be used for another purpose?

Let us try to understand the limits and tensions that face staff making the decision to share. There is a pressure on Data Protection Act principles from the way in which 'proportionality' and 'need to know' are construed in sharing information and how consent is obtained.

There is a range of conflicting legislation: the requirement to disclose in criminal cases, to disclose for legal purposes such as procurator fiscal; the 2005 Prevention of Terrorism Act and the 1991 Road Traffic Act and others each state an obligation to disclose information in certain circumstances. Specifics such as sexual disease and adverse drug reactions are collated and include demographic data about an individual.

The need to disclose information in relation to child protection, sexual abuse, and health and safety in the workplace are categorised as justifiable disclosure and there are grounds for assuming that harm may result if information is not shared. This is clear for staff as long as the concepts are well defined. However, much of the decision making takes place around the 'grey area', the 'gut feelings' and the 'niggling concerns'. Is consent required or will I go ahead and record anyway?

It is extremely difficult to provide staff with a formula of when and when not to share information. Risk assessments must be undertaken and procedures should be in place to ensure that staff are not afraid to share as they see necessary. No guidance can override the need for professional judgement, which, without strict regulation in place, still continues to be the underpinning force (DH, 2007). As long as the member of staff can justify the decision to share and ensure that risks have been assessed there should be no need to worry. Tools to support risk management such as Privacy Impact Assessment (PIA) are available and should be utilised by management when implementing policy and systems. PIA is an analysis of how information is handled (a) to ensure that handling conforms to applicable legal regulatory and policy requirements regarding privacy, (b) to determine risks of collecting information in identifiable form and (c) to examine and evaluate protections and alternative processes for handling information to mitigate potential privacy risks (Office of Management and Budget, 2003, cited in Raab et al, 2004).

An aspect of sharing is the use of language. Clearly, agreement on terminology is logical; however, it has been hard to achieve. A generic Single Shared Assessment dataset has been agreed and is generally in use across Scotland. There has also been an agreed set of definitions and standards published (Scottish Executive, 2005), which go a long way to ensuring consistent information collection. However, some anomalies still exist in practice. For instance, 'urgent' to a healthcare worker means something different to a social care worker and may have an impact on waiting times.

The confusion can be compounded where the central government departments and professional bodies all issue guidance on information sharing, which is often inconsistent. Could it be that policy development is reactionary? Consider the fast-track implementation of the 2006 Joint Inspection of Children's Services and Inspection of Social Work Services (Scotland) Act, which required 'the sharing or production of information (including medical records) for the purposes of an inspection under section 1'. This was in response to issues of disclosure raised by the medical profession where previously medical records were not made freely available.

Conclusion

Sharing information is an issue that will not go away. Despite masses of guidance, staff will still need training to ensure that they understand when it is appropriate to disclose information. Joint working opens the floodgates. The mix of cultures, professions and new situations where disclosure is requested only adds to the complexity of making it happen. If we are to maintain privacy and confidentiality of personal data handled jointly or between health and social care professionals there are a number of things we simply have to consider. The public must be able to trust the services, so efforts to maintain integrity of information are paramount. Secure databases, safe transfer of information, accurate and meaningful data, openness, honesty and transparency in policy development and enhanced understanding of the legal frameworks are essential components of joint information management.

Ultimately, the fundamental aim is to improve access to services for individual citizens. This is based on sharing appropriately information that is given in a situation of trust, and it is our duty as professional carers to ensure that information is safely kept and used.

References

6, P., Bellamy, C. and Raab, C. (2004) 'Data sharing and confidentiality: spurs, barriers and theories', Paper presented at the Political Studies Association Conference, University of Lincoln.

BASW (British Association of Social Workers) (2002) *The Code of Ethics for Social Work*, Birmingham: BASW.

Bellamy, C., Raab, C. and 6, P. (2005) 'Multi-agency working in British social policy: risk, information sharing and privacy', *Information Polity*, vol 10, nos 1-2, pp 51-63.

Cabinet Office Performance and Innovation Unit (2002) *Privacy and Data-Sharing: The Way Forward for Public Services*, London: Cabinet Office.

Commission for Healthcare Audit and Inspection (2005) *Code of Practice on Confidential Personal Information*, London: Healthcare Commission.

Consumers' Association (2003) *Consumers' Association Response to the NHS Information Authority Consultation on 'Information for Life'*, London: Consumers' Association.

Davies, S. (2001) *Taking Liberties in Confidence: A report for the Nuffield Trust on the Implications of Clause 67 of the Health and Social Care Bill*, London: London School of Economics and Political Science.

DH (Department of Health) (1997) *Report on the Review of Patient-Identifiable Information*, Caldicott Report, London: DH.

DH (2007) *Making a Difference: Safe and Secure Data Sharing Between Health and Adult Social Care Staff*, London: DH.

European Parliament (1995) *Directive 95/46/EC of the European Parliament and of the Council of 24 October 1995 on the Protection of Individuals with Regard to the Processing of Personal Data and on the Free Movement of Such Data*, Luxembourg: European Parliament.

General Medical Council (2000) *Confidentiality: Protecting and Providing Information*, London: General Medical Council.

Givens, B. (1998) *Ten Privacy Principals [sic] for Health Care*, San Diego, CA: Privacy Rights Clearinghouse.

Hawker, A. (2001) 'Privacy as an investment', *Healthcare Computing*, p 135.

Information Commissioner's Office (2006) *What Price Privacy? The Unlawful Trade in Confidential Personal Information*, Norwich: The Stationery Office.

ISO (International Standards Organization) (2005) *ISO/IEC 17799:2005: Information Technology – Code of Practice for Information Security Management*, Geneva: International Organisation for Standardisation International Electrotechnical Commission.

Kennedy, I. and Grubb, A. (1994) *Medical Law: Text with Materials* (2nd edition), London: Butterworth.

Laming, Lord (2003) *The Victoria Climbié Inquiry*, Cm 5730, London: The Stationery Office.

McLelland, R. (2006) *European Standards on Confidentiality and Privacy in Healthcare*, Belfast: Queen's University Belfast.

Moore, A. (2005) 'It's just between you and me ... and social services and police', *Nursing Standard*, vol 20, no 12, pp 14–16.

NHS Information Authority (2002) *Share with Care*, Birmingham: NHSIA.

NHS Quality Improvement Scotland (2005) *Clinical Governance & Risk Management: Achieving Safe and Effective, Patient-Focused Care. Consultation on Draft National Standards*, Edinburgh: NHS Quality Improvement Scotland.

Nursing and Midwifery Council (2004) *The Nursing and Midwifery Council Code of Professional Conduct: Standards for Conduct, Performance and Ethics* (2004), London: Nursing and Midwifery Council.

O'Brien, S., Hammond, H. and McKinnon, M. (2003) *Report of the Caleb Ness Inquiry*, Edinburgh: NHS Lothian.

Office of Management and Budget (2003) *Memorandum for Heads of Executive Departments and Agencies (OMB Guidance for Implementing the Privacy Provisions of the E-Government Act of 2002)*, Washington, DC: Office of Management and Budget.

Raab, C., 6, P., Birch, A. and Copping, M. (2004) 'Information sharing for children at risk: impacts on privacy', Edinburgh, Unpublished.

Richardson, S. and Asthana, S. (2006) 'Interagency data sharing in health and social care', *British Journal of Social Work*, vol 36, pp 657-69.

Scottish Consumer Council (2005) *Health On-Line: Public Attitudes to Data Sharing in the NHS*, Glasgow: Scottish Consumer Council.

Scottish Executive (2000a) *Report of the Joint Future Group*, Edinburgh: Scottish Executive.

Scottish Executive (2000b) *Our National Health: A Plan for Action, A Plan for Change*, Edinburgh: Scottish Executive.

Scottish Executive (2001) *For Scotland's Children: Better Integrated Children's Services*, Edinburgh: Scottish Executive.

Scottish Executive (2002) *'It's Everyone's Job to Make Sure I'm Alright': Report of the Child Protection Audit and Review*, Edinburgh: The Stationery Office.

Scottish Executive (2003a) *Partnership for Care: Scotland's Health White Paper*, Edinburgh: The Stationery Office.

Scottish Executive (2003b) *Getting our Priorities Right: Good Practice Guidance for Working with Children and Families Affected by Substance Misuse*, Edinburgh: The Stationery Office.

Scottish Executive (2003c) *NHS Code of Practice on Protecting Patient Confidentiality*, Edinburgh: Scottish Executive.

Scottish Executive (2005) *Scottish Social Care Data Standards Manual*, Edinburgh: Scottish Executive.

Scottish Executive (2006a) *Getting it Right for Every Child: Draft Children's Services (Scotland) Bill Consultation*, Edinburgh: Scottish Executive.

Scottish Executive (2006b) *Data Sharing Framework for Success Delivered*, Edinburgh: Scottish Executive.

Scottish Executive (2006c) *OpenScotland Information Age Framework*, Edinburgh: Scottish Executive.

Swain, P. A. (2006) 'A camel's nose under the tent? Some Australian perspectives on confidentiality and social work practice', *British Journal of Social Work*, vol 36, no 1, pp 91-107.

Thomas, R. (2006) *Waking Up to a Surveillance Society*, London: Information Commissioner's Office.

Conclusion

Chris Clark and Janice McGhee

Trends

The contributions to this volume demonstrate that expectations and standards defining the professional duty of confidentiality are now in an unprecedented state of flux. In an important sense there is nothing new about the obligation to safeguard individuals' privacy and therefore protect their communications with a promise of non-disclosure: it has been a key feature of the professional relationship at least since Hippocrates. But when we set this continuing obligation against the contemporary context of professional practice we see that the traditional promise, although ostensibly as highly valued as ever, is becoming increasingly problematic to interpret and to apply. What, then, has changed?

The conclusions of this book can be summarised in the following terms. At least four broad contemporary currents of change are shifting, and possibly eroding, the ethic of confidentiality between professionals and clients. It remains as vital as ever to protect individual rights and privacy, but this now has to be done by means of new and much more complex interpretations of the need to know and the right to keep silence. Personal information gathered in the course of professional practice can no longer be imagined as sealed in a locked container accessible only to the professional delivering the service and a small handful of select keyholders. Instead, we should think of personal information as located in a porous space of variable accessibility to different individuals, interests and agencies. It is the porosity that is the problem in both normative and technical senses: who should have access, and to what? And how can we make sure that a complex pattern of differential entitlement to know is actually maintained in the chaotic world of service delivery?

The first broad trend that is changing confidentiality is the increasing complexity of service delivery in the social and health services. It is driven by the discovery of new needs (or the rediscovery of old ones) and the invention of new treatments and methods of service delivery. Alongside this is the growing emphasis on the prevention and the management of current and potential future risk both to vulnerable individuals and the wider community. In the field of care for people with major disabilities, for example, reliance on the asylum as the principal model of provision has been swept away in a torrent of community-based interventions such as intensive home care, supported accommodation, new kinds of supported employment, self-advocacy and so forth. In the health services, constant new discoveries from medical research point the way to addressing hitherto intractable health problems, while new technologies open up therapies previously inconceivable. What this increasingly means is that an individual's needs will not be met by a single professional working alone – the often implicit, archetypal assumption behind the traditional ethic of confidentiality – but by complex assemblages of professionals and paraprofessionals drawn from a range of disciplines in health, social care and social control, working in several different agency structures subject to different and non-complementary modes of governance and management. Government policies to deal with this go under slogans such as 'joint working' and 'working together'. The significance of increasing service complexity for professional confidentiality has been drawn out in many of the contributions to this book. No longer is confidentiality primarily about keeping things secret: it is rather about communicating the necessary information to the appropriate people at the relevant time while preserving, as far as possible, the rights of client and family.

The second trend is the revolution in technologies for gathering and processing data. As this conclusion was written, the government was dealing with a spate of data, and public relations, disasters in which personal data on many millions of citizens had seemingly been lost in the post or by some other like mischance. Such incidents serve as useful reminders that the very possibility of personal data on 25 million people being casually sent in the post on a small plastic disc worth a few pence was inconceivable to all but the experts until very recently. More uncomfortably, we are forced to recognise that social systems for managing these hugely powerful new technologies are lagging far behind their potential for doing damage, whether inadvertently or deliberately. For social and health services the key issues are how to harness the new technologies for the good of individuals in need, and the population as a whole, while also maintaining strong safeguards for privacy and the rights of vulnerable people. It is not merely, or even most importantly, the inherent unreliability of new technologies that threatens privacy: it is much more that structures of governance and accountability have nowhere near caught up with the untamed power of new information technology. This factor is much magnified by the first trend of increasing service complexity, because joint working poses particular challenges to taming information technology. A number of contributors have also signposted the emerging use of technology in both the surveillance and support of citizens under the aegis of services, and the concomitant ethical issues this raises for practice.

The third trend concerns changing social attitudes to the concept of privacy. In every society there are broadly shared conceptions of what kind of personal information is appropriate to be shared, with whom and under what circumstances and conditions. Moral and religious teachings, and social conventions, set boundaries of what is seemly and what is shameful, what is honourable and what is disgraceful in the exposure of personal life and the disclosure of private information. It is an egregious feature of the present time that these boundaries are shifting, dissolving and reforming with different shape. Such processes are reflected in the worlds of television chat and 'reality' shows, celebrity magazines and other aspects of popular culture. Moreover, the Internet has opened up astonishing possibilities for both voluntary and involuntary self-disclosure to unprecedented numbers of unknown others. If professional confidentiality is rooted in a conception of privacy still very largely derived from the mores of 19th-century bourgeois society, it is not surprising that it is proving inadequate for the wired global village of the 21st.

A further aspect of social change is cultural pluralism. The traditional doctrine of professional confidentiality is not culturally universal; it is plainly rooted in the practice of Western medicine as it developed in the 19th and 20th centuries. In that context little weight was given to the different mores of other societies or ethnic and other minorities within Western developed countries. However, it is no longer imaginable to elaborate a professional ethic of confidentiality within the perspective of a dominant culture alone. There is a shift in theory and in values – still contentious, partial and imperfect, to be sure – away from majority ethnocentrism and towards a positive recognition of other cultural values. This raises complex issues. There can now be no automatic assumption that the mores of the majority should prevail over those of minorities. Where these may conflict it is uncertain how professionals ought to respond. For example, in the Western mainstream the rights of children have increasingly been defined and refined in such a way as to protect children's autonomy potentially against the wishes of their parents and other family members. This can seem to be at odds with cultures that differently emphasise parental authority, filial duty and obligation to the community. Professionals aiming to conscientiously protect privacy and respect confidentiality may, then, find themselves caught between unreconcilable expectations.

The fourth trend is the movement of citizens' rights from the shadows of the constitution and political theory to the glare of politics. Perhaps there was a time when British political culture was content with an assumed and largely unspoken trust in the soundness of the constitution, the good faith of political leaders, the integrity of public administration and the fairness and robustness of the justice system. Be that as it may, such trust has been replaced by the re-emergence of citizenship as the declared currency of the relationship between the individual and the state. Significantly, conceptions of citizenship have been mobilised by both liberals and libertarians anxious to protect the individual against the excessive power of the state, and socialists and communitarians anxious to use state power to improve the position of the powerless and disadvantaged. The convenient chameleon-like quality of the concept of citizenship makes it a powerful tool of rhetoric for politicians wishing to widen the appeal of their policies without appearing to sacrifice the supposed core values of their political parties.

As the debate about citizenship has shown, users of social and health services are never merely consumers but are also most certainly and necessarily eligible for the protections (and duties) of citizenship. The concept of citizenship can thus be usefully deployed to argue for, and ensure the extension of, those protections and benefits to previously relatively disempowered service users, including, for example, people with disabilities or members of minority ethnic communities. Effective strategies for equality and diversity seek the practical realisation of citizens' rights for hitherto disempowered or excluded minorities, particularly those whose cultural background, ethnicity, age, gender, sexual orientation, health status, type of ability and disability or other characteristic has rendered them particularly susceptible to a range of systemic injustices.

The right to have one's personal information properly used and applied by social and health services, and the concomitant right for that use to be properly protected by effective safeguards against unjustified, unauthorised or inadvertent disclosure, are clearly important examples of citizens' rights. These rights are now supported by legislation such as the 1998 Data Protection Act and the 1998 Human Rights Act. It is useful for professionals in the personal and health services to think of their duties in the handling of personal information as the practical counterpart of citizens' rights to privacy, protection of personal interests and entitlement to the very best service that it is possible to provide. Equally, it is obligatory for citizens to appreciate that they have a duty to consent to some of their personal information being transmitted to other parties in order to enable the best service to be provided, and to permit the protection of others or the promotion of public health in general.

Professional confidentiality reconceived: a trust-based approach

The contributions to this book show that the traditional expectations surrounding professional confidentiality are rapidly being overtaken. Nevertheless, while the practice of confidentiality is being forced to change and will need to change still more, underneath it lie enduring principles that remain valid and should continue to be observed. The following paragraphs retrace those key underlying principles that traditional confidentiality has sought to honour, and which new practices of confidentiality will equally need to implement as they respond to the trends highlighted earlier.

All the personal service professions acknowledge that human flourishing requires the highest safeguarding of personal autonomy – the capacity and right of the individual to make their own decisions by their own lights. This is the origin of the value of privacy that the professional ethic of confidentiality aimed to protect, and is a key part of the heritage of the professions from Western liberal individualism. In more recent times theorists have renewed attention to another essential for human flourishing: the need and capacity for mutual recognition and social solidarity in a web of personal relationships. The obligations arising from relationships may well compete with the aspiration to autonomy. These teachings from communitarianism, feminism, virtue ethics and other theoretical orientations thus pose a tension with the principles of privacy derived from liberal individualism.

Is the maintenance of individuals' privacy by professionals who give personal services still a viable doctrine? The professions must now be mindful that privacy is not something that can be single-mindedly given priority over other key ends. Equally important is the requirement to support and enhance those bonds and obligations of kinship and community that are essential to meeting the needs of their clients and patients. We have seen that the exact nature of these bonds will vary according to culture, social context and individual values. There is therefore no absolute or inalienable right to privacy in the arena of individuals' relationships with the social and health services. Instead, there is a range of qualified rights – qualified in the sense that the general presumption of privacy may on occasion have to give way to other rights. These include the right of vulnerable individuals to be protected from serious harm; and the right of significant persons in the social networks of individuals in need of services to have their own say in the management of difficult situations affecting their kinsperson.

Professionals are therefore in the delicate position of having to balance such competing ends both on behalf of their clients and on behalf of the general public good, to which they must also give constant attention. Recognising that professionals are asked, and empowered, to act in these ways on behalf of others, we can say, in other words, that professionals are *trustees*. A trustee is someone appointed to act on another's behalf, when the trustor is unable to make, or chooses not to make, direct decisions for themselves. A trustee may be appointed to look after matters that are too onerous or complex for the trustor to handle, or may be appointed to act when the trustor lacks full capacity, or is a child, or is dead.

The concept of professional as trustee is compatible with, but significantly enlarges, the traditional undertaking of professional confidentiality. A confidential communication is one that is given on terms of trust that the receiver will use the information for the purposes envisaged and understood by the giver of the information – and not for any other purpose, or at least not without prior consent. This is therefore a species of trustee relationship, but is circumscribed by quite limiting conditions on the range of actions open to the trustee. The enlarged concept of trusteeship is needed to take account of the many different interests that professionals, and their agencies, must now protect when they consider how to handle personal information. The reasons for this enlargement have been illustrated by all the contributions to this book, and can be summed up as follows.

Professionals continue, as they have always been, to be trustees of individuals' personal information. What the traditional ethic of confidentiality insufficiently addresses, however, is the fact that professionals are also trustees of the safety and welfare of individuals other than their immediate client, and of the wider public good. Professionals must now consciously and accountably assume this wider and more complex trusteeship role in order to answer the policy and practice concerns that have been aired in these pages. They must do so with eyes wide open to the fact that acting as trustees simultaneously to many parties, they will often have to deal with conflicting interests; and that every resolution of a conflict of interests is liable to undermine the trust of at least some of the trustors.

How, then, should professionals maximise the trust in which they are held by clients and the public, and so best fulfil the trusteeship that their role necessarily entails? Paradoxically perhaps, there is no one simple set of rules for handling personal information that will reliably support trust. On the contrary, simplistic and rigid rules are very likely to undermine trust, because they are not sensitive to the nuances of situation, relationship and context. Every citizen of advanced societies has experienced the frustration of standard and apparently reasonable bureaucratic rules producing absurd results, of which Peter Ashe's story (Chapter Nine, this volume) of anxious parents waiting for a flight arrival is a nice illustration. The essential point of a trusteeship is that the trustee is empowered with *discretion* to employ broad principles flexibly and artfully as the circumstances may seem to require – circumstances that can never be entirely foreseen or anticipated by those who place their trust in the trustee. The flip phrase, 'trust me – I'm a doctor' does nonetheless contain a truth about our relationships with professionals. We trust professionals to use their discretion in order to benefit us when we are not in a position to fully understand the multiple implications of a whole range of possible courses of actions or in situations where external constraints on actions are in place.

Rather than a simple set of rules for handling personal information, we need a set of working principles for professional policy and practice that will best conduce to trust between clients, professionals and the wider public. Such principles must encompass several problematics. A first and obvious one is that individuals have different personal values and given the opportunity, may make different choices about the handling of their personal information. Professionals need to respond to these value preferences while avoiding trespassing on the contrary legitimate preferences of others, and while avoiding arbitrariness and unfairness in the way they deal with the whole range of the client population.

The capacity for trust and the range of actions that is authorised in every trustee relationship is a function of individual agency and mental capacity. What is required for well-placed trust by children or individuals with impaired capacity will be different from what is required for well-placed trust by fully competent adults. Protecting the interests of individuals with reduced capacity for agency will mean devising trustworthy means of dealing with issues such as implied and proxy consent to particular uses of personal information and maximising their participation as citizens.

Several contributors to this book have drawn attention to the importance of cultural context and social, as opposed to purely individual, values. It is a major challenge for professional services to handle personal information in a way that respects diversity while, again, avoiding arbitrariness, inconsistency and unfairness. As trustees of personal information it falls to professionals to make reasonable and defensible decisions against a background of contradictory social and cultural values. To merit this difficult trusteeship, professionals need a high degree of sensitivity but also need to be supported by systems ensuring a high degree of public responsiveness and accountability. The importance of involving all stakeholders, including service users, in the negotiation and design of processes and systems to manage and share information is crucial to building public trust and has been highlighted by a number of contributors

Finally in this short list, working principles for sustaining trust in professionals' handling of personal information must take cognisance of the range of what is technically possible and practically feasible in record management, data sharing, privacy protection and surveillance. In essence, the availability of the new technologies for handling information means that the public is being asked to place much more trust in the good faith and competence of professionals, and in the trustworthiness of agencies and their managers to look after this information properly. As we have seen in several chapters, this is as much about ensuring that the right information is communicated to the right quarters in good time, as it is about ensuring that protected personal information does not leak out to the wrong quarters through inadvertence or intentional exploitation.

Conclusion

Professionals work within a framework of legislation, policy directives, guidance, interagency protocols and professional codes of practice. This complex maze of law, policy and practice guidance can leave professionals unclear as to what are legal and ethical approaches to sharing information and considering issues of capacity and consent. Professional practice increasingly operates in the context of 'joint working' and an environment rapidly utilising new technology, where practitioners bring differing interpretations and expectations of privacy and confidentiality. Protecting the rights of individual citizens to respect for their privacy in these conditions is, to borrow a phrase from Val Baker (Chapter Eleven, this volume), 'wonderfully complex'. The contributions to this book have begun to examine and explore some of the ethical, policy, legal and practice issues that underpin the day-to-day dilemmas and decisions arising in professional and agency practice. At the end of the day, professional judgement remains key to decision making, and it is suggested that the trust-based approach outlined above may be an effective way to begin to reframe classic issues of confidentiality and privacy in the rapidly changing landscape in social and health services.

Index

C